A HYPOCRITICAL OATH

The Problems with Our Health Care System and How to Manage Your Own Health Care Efficiently, Inexpensively and Naturally

James C Hogan

A Hypocritical Oath

First Edition 2015

All scripture references are taken from the King James Version of the Bible unless otherwise indicated.

Published by Abundant Joy Church Inc.

Copyright 2015 by Abundant Joy Church Inc.

All Rights Reserved

Contact us at jhogan222@gmail.com

Cover art by James Hogan

Printed in the United States of America

CONTENTS

1 About This Book and The Author

2 Insights About Health Care

3 Our Backwards FDA and Health Care System

4 Conventional Cancer Treatment

5 The Power of Vitamin C, Compounding and Synergy

6 Selenium

7 Coconut Oil

8 Common Sense Health care

9 Ann Jillian No More

10 Skin Cancer

11 Genetics and Cancer

12 Left for Dead

13 Colon Cancer: What I Would Do If I Had It

14 Bio-Oxidative Therapies

15 Heart Health

16 Replace or Rejuvenate

17 Mental Health

18 Pharmaceutical Hell and The Elderly

19 Aids Has Its Place in The World No More

20 The Health Care Crisis

21 Childhood Health Care

22 Other Diseases

23 The Great American Health Care Cover up

24 The Affordable Care Act

25 A Word for The Rich

26 The Great Physician

27 The Simplicity of Health Care and The Mystery of Health and Healing

28 Ebola and A Hypocritical Oath

INTRODUCTION

This is a book about health issues from a medical perspective and also from a spiritual perspective. It is not meant to be an exhaustive resource on every health issue but to give the reader a new view of health care issues by looking beyond the boundaries of the mainstream health care system. In it I discuss how you can and should take charge of your own health care, through an increase of knowledge, rather than waiting until you get sick and then leaving everything to your doctor. Also I wanted to write a book that is not too long. Something that is easy to read and reveals important truths and health facts that you can take and do further study on for your own benefit.

I believe the number one problem with the health of Americans today is the lack of knowledge and interest in health issues. In my life experiences in talking to people it amazes me how little the average person knows about taking care of their health and even more, how little they seem to care until they find themselves in a health crisis. I hope this book will spark people's interest.

In this book I not only discuss health issues from a scientific standpoint but also from a spiritual one. Since God is the creator of the body he is also the creator of everything we need for health and is also able to give us the wisdom and guidance that we need as well.

The title "A Hypocritical Oath" is a play on words. When medical doctors graduate from medical school they recite some form of the Hippocratic Oath which comes from the ancient Greek physician Hippocrates who is referred to as the father of western medicine. The oath is a promise to put the welfare of the patient first and to do them no harm. As I will show in this book, in our health care system in America today, the best and least expensive therapies are often passed over for ones that are more profitable and inferior or even harmful. I will discuss some of these therapies and natural alternatives to them.

You may not agree with everything you read in this book. You may question some things you read in this book, but I guarantee if you take the time to read it all the way through, you will learn new things you can use to improve your health, your life and the lives of other people around you. I believe you will find the information I share in this book to be, at the very least, revolutionary and life changing!

Wisdom is the principle thing; therefore get wisdom: and with all your getting get understanding. Proverbs 4:7

DISCLAIMER

In this book I speak about medical issues such as specific diseases, main stream therapies and alternative natural cures. I consider myself to be a health expert but I am not a medical doctor. I took an interest in health issues as a teenager and have been studying these issues ever since, gathering a lot of data, information and personal experiences over nearly 40 years. It all began with my father being diagnosed with high cholesterol in the early seventies. As a result, my Mother decided to begin cooking healthier and more natural food, like baking her own oatmeal bread. We even visited a local health food store, which in those days was considered to be a real oddity. They had a lot of unusual products we never saw anywhere else. Through time my family began to become very health conscious about the food we were eating for better health. As I developed an interest in sports and bodybuilding I began to become even more aware of nutrition and what I should be consuming for maximum development and benefit. Another issue that appeared on the horizon, when I was young, was the subject of cancer. As I read about cancer and saw it portrayed on television and in movies I began to question why people got cancer and why there wasn't a better way to treat it other than chemotherapy or other conventional treatments. As a result, I studied every article I ever came across on this subject and eventually found proof that there were better, safer, more natural therapies available. This also seems to be the crux of our health care crisis in America. The fact that most people don't take the time to do their own research and learn how to take care of their own bodies. Very often they leave everything up to their doctor.

In this book I share my opinions, things I have learned through study, personal experiences and things I have heard the Spirit of God say. It is the responsibility of the reader to do their own research and to consult a physician or health care professional before following any of the information I give in this book. In addition, every person's body is different in certain respects and your body's needs and responses may vary from someone else's. It takes time to learn how your body reacts to different kinds of nutrients and different kinds of exercise and stress. You are at a distinct advantage in life if you can learn as much as possible about your own body when you are well, so that if or when you become ill, you will know what to do and what not to do. You'll know what works and what doesn't. You'll be prepared to be your own best doctor. I'm not saying you shouldn't see a doctor if you have health concerns or a serious health problem. What I am saying is you'll have the knowledge you need to make wiser health decisions that can dramatically improve your quality of life and even save your life or the life of someone you know!

CHAPTER 1

ABOUT THIS BOOK AND THE AUTHOR

This book is not your average book. In it I discuss medical and scientific issues relating to the human body but I begin from a spiritual perspective.

I begin by talking about hearing the Spirit of God speak about issues of health care and healing.

This book was originally inspired by a 19-page letter I wrote back in 2011 by the same name. I felt I had an important message about our health care system that I was supposed to share with others. I emailed the original version to other pastors in December of 2011. The message of the book is the same as the original letter except that I have expanded on the original subjects.

I believe the subject of hearing God speak is a very important and relevant issue for today. Certainly there are people who would seriously question such statements or perhaps scoff or ridicule such things. Actually, even when I was a Bible college student in the mid-1980s, I was mocked by another student for stating that God spoke to me. This was in a school where we were taught that God does still speak to people today. However, over the course of time, I have come to recognize when God is speaking, whether it be through a dream, a still small voice, a momentary vision, an inward witness or even through another person's words.

There are three main criteria that I look for when a person says that God has spoken to them.

1. Is it in agreement with the teachings of Christ and the Bible as a whole?

2. Is it meant to help and to bless?

3. Does the word turn out to be accurate? Does it come to pass?

When God speaks, he speaks to help us. He speaks to warn us of danger or trouble. God desires to teach us by his Spirit, to lead us into all truth and to show us things to come.

However, when He, the Spirit of truth, has come, He will guide you into all truth; for he will not speak on His own authority, but whatever He hears He will speak; and He will tell you things to come. John 16:13. (NKJV)

However, it's up to us to take the time to earnestly seek him and to attune ourselves to spiritual things. It isn't scriptural for us to seek to hear a voice but it is scriptural to desire to be led by Gods Spirit and by His word.

In speaking to groups of people on this subject I have taken surveys to see if other people have had these kind of experiences and I have come to the conclusion that they are more commonplace than a lot of people realize. Many people have had these kind of experiences to varying degrees but they often don't acknowledge them or talk about them.

Spiritual experiences are also often subtle experiences and are often dismissed as a passing thought that is not important, or perhaps a person's own mind playing tricks on them, when in fact it's actually the Spirit of God saying something. A person may have a premonition or a dream or hear a still small voice and then just let it go and forget about it. If I believe the Spirit of God is dealing with me, I make a point of taking note of it. I usually will write it down in my journal.

Then the Lord said: Write the vision and make it plain on tablets, that he may run who reads it. Habakkuk 2:2 (NKJV)

The scriptures also tell us that there are many voices in the world and none of them without signification. If a person hears a voice speak, it's important to be able to judge that voice by the scriptures whether or not it is the Spirit of God.

Spirituality is something I was familiar with from the time I was a small child. My parents, mainly my Mother, took my brother, my sisters and I to Church regularly. I was raised Catholic as a child and the first Church I remember was a new parish called Good Sheppard. It was the 1960s, and it was where I was baptized as an infant. We met in the large basement of the new Catholic school because the main church had not been built yet. Instead of organ music they had mainly acoustic guitars with newer worship songs. There were also large modern looking fabric banners that had passages of scripture on them. The church was working to be more in step with the times of the 1960s. It was here that I first became aware of the power and presence of God. I remember as a small child sitting with my family all the way at the back of the church. It seemed like there were thousands of people there in attendance. We would sit and listen to Father Francis give his sermon and read from the scriptures. I remember feeling my heart burn within me, as the two disciples did when they were walking with Jesus on the road to Emmaus, only they didn't know it was him until later. I was only three or four years old at the time but I still remember this experience.

When I was about four years old we moved to a suburb of Milwaukee called Shorewood, because my Mother was going to be attending UW Milwaukee which was nearby. We attended a Parish there where I received my first communion. To a Christian who is not a Catholic I suppose things like child baptism and first Communion don't carry a lot of meaning. Someone may ask when did I ask Christ into my heart or when did I receive salvation? In 1971 my family moved to Menomonee Falls. When I was 12 years old I met a neighboring family that believed in the born again experience and the infilling of the Spirit. They told me I needed to be born again. Jesus spoke of this in John 3:1-8. So I went home one day and prayed a prayer for salvation. I waited to see if anything was different but nothing had seemed to change. As a result, I came to the conclusion that I already had it. One thing about the Catholic Mass, in regard to the subject of salvation, is that a confession of the Lordship of Christ is repeated at every Mass. A few years later I received adult baptism at another Church in a different town, when I was high school age.

Although spirituality was a central issue in my upbringing I was also exposed to other ideas. As I mentioned, my Mother went to college while I was still very young. She was studying for a degree in teaching, specifically in teaching emotionally disturbed and learning disabled children. She brought home text books including ones on the subject of evolution. These books had a lot of pictures and diagrams and I studied them as best I could for the age I was. As a result, I grew up believing in both the Bible and the theory of evolution. However, as I got older and into my teenage years I could see the conflict between the two beliefs systems and began to do further study. As a result, I came to the conclusion that the theory of evolution was not very scientific and that the Bible actually did contain all kinds of information supported by science, history and archeology. I found that the more the scientific world learned about the human body, matter and the universe, the more these new findings pointed to intelligent design. The design of an intelligent creator.

My parents seemed to move around a lot when I was growing up and it was always for important reasons. Either school, work or family matters like moving up north to be closer to my Grandmother after my Grandfather passed away, in the mid-seventies. My Grandmother lived in Green bay, which is where my Mother was raised as a child. My parents opted to buy an old retired dairy farm, with all of the buildings and over one hundred acres of land, just outside of Green bay, in a township called Angelica. We began a small hobby farm there with different kinds of farm animals. A few years later my Dad decided he didn't want so much land anymore so he put the place up for sale and we moved to another old dairy farm that was nicer but only had about three and half acres. It was in a place called Green Valley. I really enjoyed the beauty and quiet of being out in the country and on the farm. It was there that I was free of a lot of the trouble a young person could get into in the city. I was in a quiet place where I could become more focused on spiritual things. It was also there where we met several other Christian families who challenged us spiritually. We began to see the church world as a bigger place which included all Christian denominations. At times we were involved with Catholics and other times Assembly of God, Baptist or nondenominational Christian churches. We were even involved with spirit filled Catholic meetings.

Some of the Christian families we met, while living in the country, introduced us to well-known Full Gospel, Spirit filled Bible teachers. We began to read their books and listen to their tapes. Through them I learned more about the infilling of the Spirit and the gifts of the Spirit. At the age of 15 I received the infilling of the Spirit with little fanfare. In other words, it was not an earth shaking spiritual experience like the disciples of Jesus had on the day of Pentecost, however I began to see certain changes and gifts of the Spirit began to work in my life.

As a child it was not unusual for me to have nightmares from time to time that would cause me to wake up out of a deep sleep. However, when I received the infilling of the Spirit, I began to notice I had power over nightmares. If something bad was happening to me in a nightmare, I would often rebuke it in the name of Jesus, turning a nightmare into an over coming experience. I found I had a new degree of power working in my life. There are people who will read these comments about the infilling of the Spirit who may not relate to what I am saying. Jesus told his disciples to wait until they were endued with power from on high. They were already believers at that point. Jesus was telling them there was something more to experience in their spiritual journey.

There was additional power with signs following. I think sometimes we have to be willing to take off our denominational glasses and be willing to look beyond what we're accustomed to hearing in order to learn new things that have been in the scriptures all along.

As a teenager who desired to learn more about the Bible and spiritual things, I spent a good amount of time in prayer and studying the scriptures. I would try to get away by myself to pray in the morning or at night. When we first moved to Angelica, I would go out to do my chores in the morning and I would stop in at the old milk house to pray alone. The peace and solitude of the country seemed like the perfect place to seek and learn more about God.

As I spent time in prayer and the scriptures, issues would arise in my life where I would seek direction from God. It seemed that this was a time in my life where God didn't speak much. I think the number one way that I got spiritual direction, other than from the Bible, was from the inward witness. An inward knowing or leading that something was right or something was wrong. Later I read in a book called "How You Can Be Led by Spirit of God" by Kenneth E. Hagin, where he said he had visions of Jesus and that Jesus said to him the number one way he leads his children (after the scriptures) is by the inward witness. In other words, an inward premonition or knowing.

For as many as are led by the Spirit of God, these are the sons of God.
The Spirit Himself bears witness with our spirit that we are the children of God, Romans 8:14 and 16.

It wasn't until after I graduated from Bible College and started pastoring that I began to hear the Spirit of God speak to me from time to time and then more regularly, about issues of ministry, work and day to day life. It seemed the further I traveled down the road of Gods call upon my life, the more I became accustomed to hearing the still small voice of the Spirit directing me as to what he wanted me to do, even if sometimes it seemed almost impossible. However, in the scriptures we see that with God all things are possible.

A number of years ago, in the early 2000s, I was working in my contracting business when I heard a still small voice speak something to me. After several weeks of hearing this same phrase spoken repeatedly from time to time, I finally said to myself, "I wonder if God is trying to say something to me?" The phrase that was repeated was "Brake line, antifreeze."

I knew my work truck had an antifreeze leak and I decided to make an appointment to have a mechanic look at it and repair it. I figured there must be something going on with a break line as well. When I went back to get my truck and pay the bill, they gave me a computer printout of the work that was done. They repaired the radiator and a front brake line. God is my witness, at the top of the print out, the very top line contained only three words. They were "Break line antifreeze" the same phrase I heard repeated over and over again before I ever took my truck in to be repaired. The Spirit of God had this foresight. Over time I have had many similar experiences. One thing I found out about the leading of the Spirit and the voice of the Spirit, that I could never get away from, is that it always turned out to be right. The accuracy was disturbingly undeniable. Now that is not to say that I am perfect in everything that I do. I'm human like anyone else and I can miss it. When God speaks there is the issue of human interpretation.

Sometimes the Spirit of God will speak about things that come to pass in a short period of time. Sometimes the word may come to pass after a longer period of time, maybe even years or decades. Sometimes the Spirit of God will speak of things that can be or will be if we do certain things or do not do certain things. Some things are dependent upon our own action or in action. God, by his Spirit, endeavors to lead us to fulfill his plans and purposes for our own good and for the good of others around us. He endeavors to lead us by his Spirit for the furtherance of his Kingdom.

It is within recent times words of prophecy have become more prevalent in my life where I have begun to hear the Spirit of God speak about many different issues. This spirit of prophecy is a sign of the times as we see in the book of Joel.

And it shall come to pass afterward that I will pour out My Spirit on all flesh; your sons and your daughters shall prophecy, your old men shall dream dreams, your young men shall see visions: And also upon the servants and upon the handmaids in those days will I pour out my spirit. Joel 2:28-29

CHAPTER 2

INSIGHTS ABOUT HEALTH CARE

Over a period of years God has given me a number of dreams about the issue of health care and in recent times I have heard the Spirit of God speak on this issue. Also in recent times health care has become a major issue in our government because of the soaring costs of health care and health care insurance. When I write something I have heard the Spirit of God say, I usually will list the date that I heard it on because the date may have significance. Sometimes the word is spoken before a corresponding event occurs or sometimes the date may have some other significance. There is also the issue of seeing and knowing. When I hear a word I usually will also have insight into its meaning and write that after the word I've heard.

On 6-1-2011, I heard the Spirit of God say, "There is a Hypocritical Oath out there."

9-23-2011 "Disordinate health care system."

10-13-2011 "There are medically inept people out there." In our health care system.

When I heard these things spoken I knew what the Spirit of God was saying, since health issues have been a subject of personal interest I have studied for many years. The Spirit of God is speaking of the dysfunctional state of our health care system and medical establishment and here is the problem . . .

We Look to Our Health Care System as if It is God

The health of Americans and the state of our health care system, in regard to the treatment of disease, is disordinate because **we have forgotten God.** We look to doctors and modern medicine often before we seek the wisdom of God! **Even people of faith often think that doctors have more knowledge and wisdom than what we can receive from the creator.** This is obvious when we see the health care choices many people have made that turned out to be negative. Health care choices that did not work and/or put the patient into financial hardship or bankruptcy. People don't take the time to do their own research and then expect their doctor to know what is best. (Ultimately a person must decide what is best for themselves because the doctor will never live in a patient's body or feel what a patient feels.) Doctors often look to the medical establishment before they seek the wisdom of God. The medical establishment has become largely profit driven rather than compassion and healing driven. Over time I have found that the vast majority of people simply do not understand that modern medicine has become big business.

The problem with modern medicine, in regard to the treatment of disease in America, is it is based on the premise or presupposition that our bodies are the products of Darwinian evolution. The scriptures tell us we are the creation of God! Man says we must create new drugs to treat cancer, heart disease, HIV/AIDS, etc., for example. God says in his word that he provided everything we would need when he first placed man in the Garden of Eden. **We should make health care as simple and as uncomplicated as possible!**

(A brief note about Darwin. When Charles Darwin wrote his book about his theory, The Origin of the Species, he had no knowledge about the complexity or inner workings of the human cell, for example. With the advent of high powered microscopes, science has discovered how individual cells function. If Darwin knew then, what microbiologists know now, perhaps he would not have held the same views. Science has discovered that the inner workings of an individual human cell are like a high tech modern day factory. In other words, something as simple and basic as a human cell is so complex in its internal functions, one must conclude it's too complex to have come about by chance. Actually Darwin did comment about another part of the body, the human eye, where he said it seemed absurd to believe it could have evolved by natural selection. When you read his comment in context it seems he was sending a mixed message about the theory of evolution. He thought it was absurd and yet somehow plausible. To me that is a confusing message.)

What We Need

In the world of science, we have learned that there are specific things our bodies need to function and to stay healthy.

Fresh air (sufficient oxygen)

Water (pure water)

Food (which includes specific nutrients such as proteins, fats, carbohydrates,
fiber, vitamins and minerals, bioflavonoids, polyphenols, probiotics, etc.)

Exercise

Sleep

Sunlight

Healthy human relations

Prayer

Another key is we need these things in **balance!** Too much or not enough of the things we need for life can bring about serious health problems and can lead to disease! In fact, scientific studies have revealed that a deficiency in a single key nutrient can lead to disease and even death! Other things can lead to disease as well, such as too many toxins in the body and too much stress.

Health care, in the simplest terms, is maintaining balance in healthy diet and lifestyle choices! Our bodies require special care for health and longevity. Studies show that there is a large percentage of Americans who are in a state of perpetual constipation, dehydration and malnutrition due to eating the wrong foods, drinking the wrong beverages, not getting enough exercise and proper sleep. What we need is a diet that contains plenty of fresh fruits, nuts, vegetables and healthy whole grain foods. Foods that have lots of dietary fiber, polyphenols, antioxidants and living enzymes. Foods that cause our bodies to maintain a healthy ph level where the body is not acidic. Ideally we should have some foods that still have living microbes on it from healthy living soil, to promote proper function of the colon. Also we need foods that are raised responsibly, that are not laden with chemical pesticides, herbicides, and fertilizers. These things create toxicity in our bodies. In other words, we need to get back to the way things used to be before processed, unhealthy, low nutrient food came into being.

In the early 1900s, with the advent of synthetic nitrogen fertilizer and other modern farming methods, farmers were able to produce more food faster than ever before. However, what most people didn't realize then, and many don't realize even today, is that with these new modern farming methods our modern culture sacrificed quality for quantity. Farmers started producing more food but food with a lower nutrient level and of a lower quality. These modern farming methods also began to have an impact on the environment as well.

In the early 1900s, a young chiropractor by the name of Forest Shaklee began working on techniques for extracting nutrients from food and began producing an early version of the vitamin pill. He found that if you take a piece of fruit, for example, and take away the water, fiber and carbohydrate, the remaining substances left are the vitamins, minerals and bioflavonoids. He also discovered that modern farming practices produced food high in calories but low in nutrients. Feeding this type of grain to pigs and other livestock yielded large animals that had less meat and more fat. These new modern farming methods, which depended on synthetic chemicals, also had a negative effect on the condition of the soil that was being farmed. Soil in the fields of farms using these new methods was becoming harder and lifeless. Soil with less and less microbes, living organisms and nutrients normally found in healthy soil.

Today you can walk into most grocery stores and find some foods that are labeled as organic. This means the food was raised naturally without chemical fertilizers, herbicides or pesticides. With organic foods you are getting something that has not had its growth chemically stimulated. Some people will say there isn't much difference between organic and non-organic food. Actually there are some very real differences. With organic you are getting food that has no synthetic chemical residue in or on it. Food that required healthy, living, nutrient rich soil to achieve its normal growth without chemical fertilizers. This means per calorie you are getting more nutrition without adding chemical toxins to your body. You are getting a food that is pure with a greater nutritional density. However, the nutritional content of the food is also directly dependent on the fertility or nutrient content of the soil.

This brings us to the subject of cellular integrity. Foods that are grown organically have a higher cellular integrity than non-organic. This means the food is of a higher quality. To prove what I'm saying is true, take an organic tomato or an organic cantaloupe or some other organic food and put it in your refrigerator alongside the same food that is non-organic. I have found that organic foods usually last longer before spoiling. Sometimes they last a lot longer. You know the old saying, you are what you eat. The cellular integrity of the food you eat has a direct effect on the cellular integrity of your own body.

I realize not everyone can afford to eat all organic but there are some very important dietary changes anyone can make when they are informed about the importance of consuming whole foods rather than processed foods. I believe, along with many health experts, that the advent of modern farming and mass production of processed foods, throughout the twentieth century, is the main cause of most of the diseases people suffer from today in industrialized countries.

The Importance of Proper Hydration

We also need to be properly hydrated. We need pure water that does not contain chlorine and other contaminants. There are so many chemicals and contaminants in the environment today, including naturally occurring ones like arsenic for example. The only way you can be sure the water you are drinking is really pure is by either purifying it or getting it from a source that is regularly analyzed that shows it is pure. There are many kinds of water purifiers out there and they all have varying degrees of effectiveness. I believe distilled water is the purest. Reverse osmosis is also very effective. Ozonation is very effective in killing microorganisms but doesn't remove chemicals or sediment. Some purification systems use several different stages to filter and purify and are very effective. If you buy bottled water at the store, take the time to read the label to see exactly what kind of water it is. Some bottled water hasn't had anything done to it at all and therefore could be exactly the same as your own tap water, containing a lot of things you don't want. Water is the number one compound of all living things. It is the number one surfactant or cleansing agent in the world. By it nearly everything is transported in and out of the body. Water cannot do the job it was intended to do if it is carrying pollutants into your body. Truly pure water not only makes it possible for your body to be properly hydrated but to detoxify as well. Pure water, free of chemicals and toxins is an absolute necessity for optimal health.

Recently I did an in depth study of the health effects of distilled or purified water. I found a long list of doctors that attest to its ability to flush unwanted minerals and toxins out of the body thus curing many different health problems such as arthritis, kidney stones, sciatica, atherosclerosis and many others. Alexander Graham Bell swore by its benefits. One doctor did a long term study of people who drank rain water before municipal water systems came into being, verses those who drank well water or municipal water. He found the ones that drank pure rain water experienced much better health. I only read one comment made by one doctor who said distilled water shouldn't be used over a long period of time because it can remove vital minerals from the body. There are other doctors who do not agree with that. I don't know if that's true, however I've been drinking purified or distilled water for such a long time I decided to temporarily switch to natural spring water just to experience the difference. One thing I do know is that I've been drinking purified water for such a long time that I can immediately tell the difference if I drink water from a municipal water supply. If a municipal treatment system is not very good or adds a noticeable amount of chlorine, one glassful will cause my digestive system to begin shutting down.

As I said before, there is no way for you to know what is actually in your water from day to day unless it is regularly analyzed or it is purified by an effective purification system. This is particularly true of municipal or city water where there can be unknown factors in the daily treatment system and in the condition of the endless miles of pipes. Also the human body was not made to consume chlorine. I read one study that showed people who drank water from a chlorinated municipal water supply over their lifetime had a 30% higher rate of bladder cancer. You cannot maximize health by drinking chlorinated and fluoridated water that contains who knows how many other contaminants. Clearly we are fortunate to have the available water supply that we have here in American cities compared to third world nations. However, to truly have healthy water, we are going to have to take the extra step of point of use purification if we're going drink tap water regularly. In addition to consuming healthy water it's also important to note that the water we bath and shower in also can affect our health and appearance. If you shower with water that contains a lot of minerals, chemicals and other impurities, those things will not only leave a residue on your skin and hair but some will also be absorbed into the body through the skin. This is why I recommend finding a good multistage shower filter or whole house water system filter so you don't end up leaving a lot of residue and contaminants on your skin every time you bath or shower. You'll feel healthier and look healthier as a result. If you're on well water, I recommend having your water analyzed every year or every few years. At the very least have it analyzed for bacteria, nitrates and arsenic. You can take the sample yourself and send it into a lab or you can hire a professional to do it.

We also need healthy living and work environments that are not full of toxins, which is a subject I speak more on later in the book.

In the study of indigenous people groups, from places in the world that still have their traditional native diets, western diseases are virtually unknown. We need to look at what they are doing right and follow their example! I'm not talking about extreme diets but basic common sense about what we eat and how we live. Eating and living in a more healthful and natural way.

Our health care establishment is making the issue of health care complicated and we are missing the forest for the trees. We need to get back to the basics of things people knew years ago and discoveries about health that have been made but brushed aside for the latest drugs being marketed by the pharmaceutical industry.

The Snow Ball Effect

In the treatment of disease, our health care system is suffering from the snow ball effect. A greater and greater emphasis is put on the intervention of medical science from the standpoint of drugs and surgery and the population is getting sicker and more dependent upon a system of "sick care" rather than health care. Our for profit health care system lacks proper government oversight (or maybe public non-government oversight) and has become like a runaway train. Our health care system has become largely profit driven rather than healing driven. I truly believe that the lack of wise oversight by our government, over the decades since the FDA was established, has cost the American people possibly trillions in unnecessary health care costs, and loss of productivity, not to mention the suffering and loss of life!

CHAPTER 3

OUR BACKWARDS FDA AND HEALTH CARE SYSTEM

Recently I was reading a disclaimer on a bottle of Vitamin C I bought. It says . . .
*This statement has not been evaluated by the Food and Drug Administration. This product is not intended to diagnose, treat, cure or prevent any disease.
I noticed all of my nutritional supplements have this statement on the label. I noticed that the over the counter drugs I have in my medicine cabinet do not have this statement on their labels.
Vitamin C is the only cure for scurvy! It is necessary for many biological functions in the body including the proper function of the immune system. It is a necessary nutrient. How is it possible the Food and Drug Administration, of a nation like the United States of America, would require a disclaimer on Vitamin C and other necessary nutrients that are proven to be the only cure for certain diseases? However, they don't require the same labeling for chemical medicines that only temporarily treat symptoms and can leave you with serious side effects? Drugs do have safety labeling but the difference between the two implies

that nutritional supplements have no proven value. It doesn't make sense! It is illogical! The real issue is the interests of the pharmaceutical industry and their influence with the FDA, which I'll talk about more later.

CHAPTER 4

CONVENTIONAL CANCER TREATMENT

Over the years our health care establishment has been waging a war on cancer. Billions of dollars have been spent on research and development of new drug therapies for different kinds of cancer. There have even been many fund raising events where well-meaning people have given of their own money to help find a cure. Yet cancer still kills more than 500,000 Americans every year. The National Institute of Health (NIH) estimated 585,720 Americans would die of cancer in 2014, on average almost 1600 people per day. More people are being diagnosed with some type of cancer than ever before in history. I recently read in one article that 1 in 4 Americans will be diagnosed with some form of cancer in their life time. The annual cost for cancer care in the U.S estimates can vary greatly depending on the source of the information. The NIH estimates overall costs of cancer in 2009 were $216.6 billion. Some others sources estimate the current annual cost to be much higher. However, statistics show on average, that people who are diagnosed with cancer and **do not** receive conventional cancer treatment such as chemotherapy, radiation or mutilating surgery, (removal of body parts) actually live longer than those that do receive such treatments! There have been a number of in depth studies done over time, beginning back as early as 1843 and studies done in recent years that reveal the harm and failure of conventional cancer treatment and also the high cost of it.

Here is a statement I have found over and over again in many different articles on the subject alternative cancer treatments. Dr. Hardin Jones, professor of medical physics and physiology at the University of California Berkeley said, "My studies have proven conclusively that untreated cancer victims actually live up to four times longer than treated individuals. For a typical type of cancer, people who refused treatment lived for an average of 12-½ years. Those who accepted surgery or other kinds of treatment (chemotherapy, radiation, cobalt) lived an average of only three years…I attribute this to the traumatic effect of surgery on the body's natural defense mechanism. The body has a natural defense against every type of cancer."

In addition to the aforementioned quote I personally have heard Oncologists and nurses say that the use of chemotherapy is a race against time once it has begun. The number one reason being the negative impact of chemotherapy on the body. Often times the question is what's going to kill you first, the chemo or the cancer? In more recent times chemotherapy has become more specific in targeting different kinds of cancer and perhaps not always as quickly toxic as it was 30 or 40 years ago, but the long term effects and outcomes are still very similar.

Recently (as of January 2014) I found a website for Envita Medical Centers. I found statements made about the ineffectiveness of chemotherapy such as "Why are 70% of Cancer Patients Unresponsive to Chemotherapy Treatments?" In the year 2014 only 30% of cancer patients seem to be responding to chemotherapy? Also what about the negative side effects of chemotherapy and the 5 and 10-year survival rates? **What other things in our society are considered acceptable that have a 70% failure rate and cost as much as chemotherapy and also have the negative side effects?** It's what you could call a triple whammy! It has a 70% failure rate, it's very expensive and it may kill you! Knowing these facts would definitely make me look elsewhere for another kind of treatment. With the number of people who are still dying from cancer it sounds like main stream medicine is failing miserably in its battle against cancer. If the FDA and the surgeon General were to act on the statistical success rate of conventional cancer treatments here in the U.S, as opposed to more natural alternative approaches, conventional cancer treatments would be outlawed and considered fraud! And they should be, in my opinion!

The statement from Envita was to point out that chemotherapy should be more customized to target specific kinds of cancer for better results, in their opinion, which of course I do not agree with.

When an individual is diagnosed with cancer, often times they are told they must begin chemotherapy immediately. The real issue a doctor should focus on is what is causing this condition? **Cancer is not just a disease, it is a symptom of a larger problem.** Something is causing the body to be out of balance biochemically. There may be one or a combination of different causes, such as nutritional deficiency, toxicity, and or stress.

In 1923 German biochemist Dr. Otto Warburg discovered that cancer occurs in cells that are deprived of 60% of their normal oxygen requirements and then a process of fermentation takes place in the cell to produce its energy because of a lack of oxygen. When this occurs the normal process of cell replication is altered and a cell can begin to replicate in an uncontrolled manner. In 1931 Dr. Warburg was awarded the Nobel Prize for his discoveries in cancer research.

Another factor that may play a role in cancer is a combination of toxicity and free radical damage to the cell. It's seems clear that the replication mechanism in the DNA of the cancer cell has been altered or damaged, thus uncontrolled replication.

One hypothesis Dr. Warburg had about the formation of cancer cells is that certain bad bacteria, that had been allowed to grow in the body, may have created a buildup of plaque on cell walls, thus blocking proper oxygen flow into the cells. I believe that the simplest answer to this problem would be proper immune function and or medical intervention that assists and mimics natural immune function. White blood cells produce hydrogen peroxide. Hydrogen peroxide is the great universal cleansing agent of the body after water. It has the power to safely remove plaque and destroy every viral and bacterial infection if it's in a strong enough concentration in the body. Certain natural nutritional supplements such as vitamin C and selenium can dramatically boost immune response within a short period of time. Hydrogen peroxide can also be administered to the body in a number of different ways such as orally or intravenously. Another positive effect of added hydrogen peroxide is that as it reacts and dissipates it also increases oxygen levels in the body. Ozone therapy also increases hydrogen peroxide and oxygen levels in the body.

In recent years an Italian oncologist, Dr. Tullio Simoncini, concluded that the white fungus candida, which has been known for a long time to be present in cancerous tumors, may actually be the cause or partial cause of the development and spread of cancer in the body. This idea seems to go hand in hand with Dr. Warburgs theory of something present in the body that prevents oxygen from getting to cancer cells. Dr. Tullio focused on using targeted baking soda treatments to cure cancer with a high level of success.

There are many excellent books and resources currently available on the subject of alternative cancer treatments verses conventional. I have found many articles written by Doctors and other experts on the internet such as Natural News, Family Health News, Democracy Now, GAP, Info Wars, Dr. Julian Whitaker, Mercola.com and many others. I would also like to encourage you to look up the books "The Politics of Healing" by Daniel Haley and "Questioning Chemotherapy" by Dr. Ralph Moss. You will discover shocking facts and true stories about what really goes on in our health care system. You can also find in depth articles about these and other similar books online. If you don't use the internet you can find these books and articles at many health food stores and book stores.

CHAPTER 5

THE POWER OF VITAMIN C, COMPOUNDING AND SYNERGY

My first introduction to vitamins, that I can remember, was when I was a teenager in the mid to late 1970's when some neighbors introduced my family to Shaklee products. This was a good introduction because of Dr. Forest Shaklee's pioneering work with vitamins. The one thing that was unique about Shaklee vitamin C was the fact that it contained a lot more than just vitamin C (ascorbic acid). It contained a large amount of active bioflavonoids from fruit peel, rose hips, rutin and hesperidin. Forest Shaklee understood the importance of bioflavonoids that occur in nature with vitamins and he understood the power of synergy. Since that time many vitamin companies are now doing the same thing and I personally use a variety of nutritional products from different companies.

Another strong proponent of vitamin C use was the famous biochemist and Nobel Prize winner Linus Pauling who is considered to be one of the most important chemists in history. He is the only person who has ever received two unshared Nobel Prizes, one in chemistry and one for peace. Because of his own health issues and because of the influence by other scientists who were studying nutritional science, Pauling began to study vitamin C and eventually became a proponent of taking large doses of vitamin C. He recommended it for general health and the use of oral and intravenous vitamin C for cancer patients. Pauling was convinced of its effectiveness even though he received a lot of criticism from those in conventional medicine. He continued to take large doses until he died at age 93. However, amidst all of the criticism he received from those in conventional medicine, it's interesting to note that there are many oncologists who believe intravenous vitamin C is better than chemotherapy. Many doctors are aware of the fact that Vitamin C doesn't have the negative side effects of chemo but actually does a lot of opposite things such as boost the immune system and increase production of hydrogen peroxide in the blood. The problem is vitamin C is usually not in the protocol of treatments used in treating disease, in conventional medicine, because it's not a patentable drug that can create a lot of profit.

    I first used Shaklee 500 milligram sustained release vitamin C as a teenager for things like colds and flues. Over time I have used a number of different brands of vitamin C including brands that have no other additional ingredients like bioflavonoids. In experimenting with different kinds of vitamin C to fight different kinds of infection I have had some very dramatic experiences that I learned from. One thing I found out is that some vitamin brands or formulations can produce powerful results while some others don't seem to do anything. I discovered that a quality vitamin C supplement with bioflavonoids, taken in the right quantity, can kill an infection within hours! I also found, that in comparison, vitamin C alone is not nearly as effective.

During the winter in early 1999 I contracted a throat infection that became so bad, within a short period of time, I decided to go to urgent care to see if I had strep throat. I tried gargling and throat sprays and it just seemed to get worse until it felt like my throat was beginning to swell up. The doctor told me he didn't see any signs of strep but he did prescribe an antibiotic. The downside was that I was in a lot of pain and was told it would take several days for the antibiotic to work. Several days is a long time when you are in pain every time you swallow. As I was driving home I remembered I had a bottle of Shaklee vitamin C in the kitchen cupboard. When I got back I took about 3.5 grams at one time and then a few more 500 milligram tablets every few hours. To my amazement, within a couple of hours, I was about 80% better and finally conquered the infection completely within a couple of days. To a person who has had sore throats and other infections before, this was an undeniably dramatic result. I opted not to use the antibiotics.

Another unusual experience I had with using vitamin C happened about 14 years ago on a trip to Barbados. I picked up a bad cold infection, I believe I caught on the plane, on my way there. Even though the weather was warm and sunny every day, I had developed a runny nose that ran nonstop. After trying several cold medications that didn't do anything, I decided to look for a health food store where I could buy a quality vitamin C supplement. I found a vitamin C product made by Natural Factors from Canada that contained a lot of bioflavonoids. God is my witness, as soon as I walked out the door of the mall, in my hopeful expectation to end my misery, I opened the bottle and the moment the tablet touched my tongue my runny nose dried up! It stopped running like you snapped your fingers! Perhaps I had this unusual experience because the Spirit of God wanted to teach me something about the power of vitamin C.

As I have described, there is power and synergy when certain nutrients are combined and taken at the same time, where you can get a much greater effect than if the different nutrients were taken alone. Unfortunately, I think this is a concept Linus Pauling didn't understand in his early years of studying vitamin C. It is something Forest Shaklee understood and pioneered early on.

CHAPTER 6

SELENIUM

It has been known for a long time that cancer rates have been higher in people and cattle in parts of the world where there is selenium deficiency in the soil, such as certain parts of China and Australia for example. Selenium is an essential mineral and a powerful antioxidant. In Australia, sheep and cattle ranchers regularly supplement their herds with selenium to prevent cancer and white muscle disease. Selenium is a key nutrient required for proper cell function and immune function. There have been cases where cancer has been shown to be reversible just by supplementing with sufficient amounts of selenium!

Selenium deficiency is a perfect example of how the imbalance of a single nutrient can cause disease and death!

In chapter 13 I include further information on the vital role of selenium.

In the year 2016, our health care system should be better, more effective and more advanced than ever before in history. Doctors should be capitalizing on all of the past wisdom, knowledge and experience of those that have gone before them. If this was the case, then doctors would first run a series of tests and ask questions about diet and lifestyle to determine what is causing the biochemical imbalance in the body that has produced cancer and other disease as well.

A doctor that is wise and compassionate would advise the patient to begin certain lifestyle and dietary changes. These changes would be aimed to bring the body back into a place of nutritional and biochemical balance, boost immune function and increase oxygen levels in the body. By taking these actions cancer could be reversed quickly, and has been for many. Why? Because the creator designed the body with a powerful capacity to heal itself. God also created natural organic compounds in nature, which are recognized by the body, that work in harmony with the body's natural healing processes!

The body has been created to heal itself when provided with the proper care and nutrients!

The problem with conventional cancer treatments is that they work against the natural healing processes of the body. Conventional cancer treatments suppress and damage the immune system as well as other organs, eventually making it impossible for the body to fight back and recover in many cases. Thus the low survival rates beyond five and ten years. In my lifetime I have met many people who have been through chemotherapy and they have explained to me in detail the long term negative effects it has had on their immune system and overall health. **These treatments of poisoning, burning and dismembering should remind us more of the medieval battles and torture of the dark ages rather than modern medicine.** It seems clear that there are certain aspects of our health care system that are still operating in the dark ages!

It is interesting to note that the majority of oncologists surveyed, in one article I read, said that if they or a family member had cancer, they would use alternative therapies they believe are more effective and safer than chemotherapy such as intravenous vitamin C.

What does this say about the current state of our health care system? It says there is something seriously wrong! Shouldn't an oncologist prescribe the best therapy or treatment known? It seems the pharmaceutical companies that manufacture chemotherapy drugs and the doctors that administer them and other conventional cancer treatments, function without any human compassion or conscience toward their fellow man! They're following the status quo without questioning the system and without challenging it, while many of these heath care professionals know there are better options out there.

Part of the problem is that the Federal Government seems to be unable to deal with this kind of abuse and fraud in our health care system. Perhaps this reveals how the hierarchy of corporate America has corrupted and influenced our government. The FDA should have dealt with these kind of issues long ago but it seems clear the influence from the medical and pharmaceutical establishments has been too great for significant change to occur! Some have stated that the FDA was actually established for the purpose of protecting the interests of large corporations rather than that of the American public!

In recent times there has been some positive change in the FDA due to whistle blowers like Dr. David Graham, who brought to light the failure of the approval process of the blockbuster drug Vioxx and other dangerous drugs. However, there is much more that needs to be done. I would like to encourage you to read Dr. David Grahams full story on websites such as GAP (Government Accountability Project) and view his interview on the Television program NOW that aired on PBS on October 21st 2005. There is also a short segment on You Tube titled "The FDA is there to serve the drug industry, not the public says Dr. David Graham of the FDA."

This is a perfect example of why our government is so deeply in debt. The government is failing to protect "We the people" from tyranny and fraud in the corporate world! **Corporate powers that function without conscience or care for the people, are literally bleeding our nation and the common wealth of the people dry!** It is no wonder our health care system has been spiraling toward a financial and economic crisis in recent years!

Because our health care system is a for profit system that is so loosely monitored by the Government, there are many surgical procedures and drug therapies that are used, more often than not, just to create cash flow and profits for the companies, hospitals and doctors that use them. There have been many studies that have documented this fact. Dr. Julian Whitaker, on his website, cites a study done on heart bypass surgery patients and explains that the vast majority of individuals that have heart bypass surgery did not actually need it. Measurement of their heart function before surgery revealed that heart bypass surgery was unwarranted!

Recently a news report came out about a Michigan Doctor, Dr. Farid Fata, who gave unnecessary cancer treatments to 553 patients. Prosecutors are seeking a 175 year prison sentence. Dr. Fata was arrested in 2013 for health care fraud. I would like to encourage you to look up and read the details of this case and how people's health was damaged by the unnecessary treatments Dr. Fata administered to his patients who placed implicit trust in him, their doctor.

What can be done to change this? Our Government needs a board of health care experts that are not from the conventional medicine mind set, and who are not from corporate America. Whose function is to promote the most effective and economical health care choices and to also pinpoint those that are harmful. Individuals such as medical doctors who have openly spoken out about the problems in our current system and have demonstrated they have real solutions that work. Individuals that possess the wisdom of God. Change would also occur if the Surgeon General and the FDA would begin to take appropriate action along these lines.

CHAPTER 7

COCONUT OIL

Coconut oil was once considered unhealthy because of its high saturated fat content but in recent years it has gained new popularity in the health food industry due to new research and facts that have come out about it. It's now considered a super food because of all of the health benefits associated with it. It is also touted by many nutritional experts to be the healthiest oil or fat you can consume. Several things that are unique about coconut oil is that most of the saturated fatty acids are medium chain triglycerides which are quickly assimilated by the body, which actually help improve metabolism and energy. Another is that it is a solid below 76 degrees Fahrenheit and turns into a liquid above that, which means it will always remain a liquid in the body and will not damage the arteries like some other fats. As a result, you can easily use it as a replacement for lard, butter, or hydrogenated vegetable shortening in cooking or baking. I use it in my cooking and baking and have found it increases energy without adding any fatty weight gain.

Health experts recommend using virgin, organic coconut oil for the best health benefits. They note that many indigenous people groups around the world have used coconut as a staple in their diets for thousands of years and have only had positive health benefits associated with it. Here are some of the health issues that the benefits of coconut oil have been used for.

Heart and cardiovascular health

Improved metabolism, energy, strength and weight loss

Skin and hair care

Immunity against infections

Candida

Alzheimer's and Dementia

Diabetes

And many other health issues.

Currently I'm experimenting with taking a level teaspoon several times a day. In its solid form it's easy to take orally all by itself. Some people will add it to their coffee or tea which I don't particularly care for. Be careful of using too much at one time since it is a natural laxative if taken in a large enough amount, like several tablespoons. I would like to encourage you to take the time to do further personal research on the many health benefits and uses of coconut oil.

There are also many other sources of healthy oils and fats found in nature including virgin olive oil, salmon, sardines, flaxseeds, walnuts, almonds, avocados, egg yolks and many other sources. Consuming the right amount of fat is a necessary part of a healthy diet and is required for the proper assimilation of the food you eat.

CHAPTER 8

COMMON SENSE AND HEALTH CARE

For many years now it has become common advice for a person to get a second and even a third opinion when considering treatment or surgery for a medical condition. What this means is that not every doctor is the same. Not every doctor has the same knowledge or expertise. It also means you as the patient have to make a personal judgment. It means you are actually beginning to do your own research on the subject so you as the patient can make a well informed, intelligent decision about your own health. Doing your own research and using common sense in your health care decisions can go a long way toward a better, healthier future. Take for example the issue of cancer and chemotherapy. I remember even as a young person in my teenage years, that I seriously questioned the use of chemotherapy to treat cancer. Why? Because the treatment seemed to be worse than the disease! What does common sense tell you about chemotherapy when you see a person become so ill after their treatment that they are sick to their stomach? That they have to vomit and they can't eat anything for a while or their appetite has been dramatically reduced? What does it tell you about chemotherapy when a person begins to lose their hair and then eventually go completely bald? Or when a patient becomes pale, sickly and weak? **It reveals that chemotherapy is not good medicine.** It's not working in harmony with the body. All of the side effects of chemotherapy are consistent with the symptoms a person has when they have been poisoned! Chemotherapy does not just poison cancer cells, it also poisons the entire body. Poisoning is the reason why a patient's immune system becomes dramatically suppressed during chemo and why a patient can become sick from any infection that comes along while on chemotherapy. Poisoning is also the reason why former cancer patient's immune systems may never be the same again after having chemotherapy treatments.

Over the years I have met many people who have been diagnosed with cancer. People I have known personally and people I have just met in passing. Actually for a period of time I worked as a volunteer Chaplain in a cancer ward of a nearby hospital. There are three consistent themes that I have heard over and over again. The first are individuals who made the decision to go with chemotherapy. In talking to these people about their cancer treatment it has been common for these people to tell about the negative impact the cancer treatment had on their bodies. In addition, if they did not have sufficient health insurance, they also had a large medical bill they had to pay off as well.

The second group are those who had chemotherapy and were not only adversely affected by it but ended up dying within a few months or years later.

The third common theme is that of those who were diagnosed with cancer but they opted against conventional cancer treatments. They decided to make changes to their diet and lifestyle. To begin to eat and live in a much more health conscious way so their body would be able to correct and heal itself. The difference between this group and the first and second is that they didn't have any of the negative side effects of the conventional cancer treatments and they didn't have any giant medical bills!

About 20 years ago I was at a Christian singles retreat being held at a conference center in Green Lake. It was right on Green Lake in a beautiful, relaxing wilderness setting. I had just walked outside after one of the conference sessions when I struck up a conversation with a lady who was walking the same direction I was. Somehow we got on the subject of health and cancer. She shared her personal story with me of how a number of years prior she had been diagnosed with uterine cancer. She related to me how the doctor advised her she must begin chemotherapy immediately. However, she had an inner premonition not to do it. She said she had this inner sense that if she took the chemotherapy she would die. As a result, she decided against the doctor's advice for conventional cancer treatment and began eating an all-natural vegetarian and organic diet. She said she was now cancer free for several years and in great health! This is a reoccurring story I have heard many times over. People using common sense and taking charge of their own health. In addition, these people also had a gut sense, and inner intuition of what to avoid. This is what we need from God. We need to learn to pray for wisdom and guidance from Gods Spirit in our life's decisions. We also need to take time to learn. We need to take the time to do our own research and to learn before we make the decision to take the advice of conventional health care or do something alternative.

CHAPTER 9

"ANN JILLIAN NO MORE"

On **9**-12-11 I heard the Spirit of God say, "Ann Jillian no more."

I remember hearing years ago that Ann Jillian, who starred in the 1980s sitcom, It's a Living, was diagnosed with breast cancer and underwent treatment which included a double mastectomy. She later starred in a movie about her own life story, The Ann Jillian Story. Years later, in the early 90s I was listening to a Christian radio station and heard an interview with a Medical Doctor by the name of Doctor Lorrain Day. I learned that she had appeared on nationally televised talk shows and news programs and was internationally known. She shared her story of being diagnosed with breast cancer and how she beat cancer without conventional treatments. She did have a large tumor surgically removed but refused chemo, radiation and mastectomy surgery. She shared her ten step program to getting well and how she made a full recovery through healthy dietary and lifestyle changes. She explained that having body parts surgically removed was not the solution to beating cancer, which I agree with. I would like to say I do not necessarily agree with everything she teaches but she was successful with her program and many others have also been successful with her program or similar programs that focus on vegan, whole natural foods and positive, healthy lifestyle changes.

In this writing I am not criticizing anyone who has opted to have any kind of cancer treatment. I know that Ann Jillian, in her life, has given a lot of her time to the cause of breast cancer awareness. Since her experience with cancer many more women, including women who are in the public eye, have gone through the same thing. It seems there is a growing and alarming trend toward mastectomy surgery. What the Spirit of God is saying is that conventional cancer treatments, such as the removal of body parts, is not necessary and is not the solution to treating cancer. (A person's life can be saved by removing a cancerous body part but wouldn't it be better to solve the cancer problem and save important body parts?) Ultimately the responsibility for this trend lies with our current medical establishment that has failed to offer better solutions. As Dr. Lorrain Day explains in her video series, Cancer Doesn't Scare Me Anymore, there is a better way. God has provided the cure to this disease within our own bodies and within nature! All types of cancer can be reversed through specific lifestyle and dietary changes. Through these changes the body has the power to heal itself and eradicate all cancer.

As with everything I say in this book, I encourage you to take the time to do your own research. If you do not use the internet you may want to take the time to learn how. One way is to go to your local library and ask the librarian to show you the basics. With the internet you can search out a lot of information in a very small amount of time and you can print it out if you like. You don't have to learn how to use the internet If you so choose but I use it a lot for my own research. Also, in dealing with disease, take time to get different opinions from health professionals including homeopathic professionals. Take time to do your own research. Take time to pray over your situation to get wisdom from the Spirit of God and the Word of God. God has all the answers because he is the one that created our bodies!

CHAPTER 10

SKIN CANCER

There is one type of cancer that I would recommend adding an additional step of treatment beyond dietary and lifestyle changes and that is skin cancer. Skin cancer is currently the most common type of cancer. According to the American Cancer Society more than 3.5 million (non-melanoma) skin cancers are diagnosed each year in the United States and more than 76,000 cases of melanoma (the most serious form of skin cancer) were expected to be diagnosed in 2014. That's more than all other cancers combined. They also say skin cancer has been on the rise over the past few decades. I think a lot of people are unsure of how much exposure to the sun is safe. There are a lot of different thoughts out there on this subject. I think everyone understands that we all need a certain amount of sunshine for health. Sunshine causes our bodies to produce vitamin D, serotonin and is related to many other positive health effects. However, if you get too much, you can get sunburn, skin damage and eventually may develop some form of skin cancer.

When my father was young he had a lot of exposure to the sun and had numerous sun burns. In recent years he has had a number of small areas that were diagnosed as cancer or precancerous. Some spots were freeze treated some were surgically removed. Some people have a naturally greater resistance to skin cancer than others, particularly people who originated from hotter climates who have darker skin. However, no matter who you are, I think the most important issue is avoid staying out in the sun for too long. Allow your skin to adjust over a period of time without getting burned. I read one study that showed that people whose work requires them to work outside have lower incidences of skin cancer than those who work inside. In other words, their skin has become accustomed to regular exposure over a period of time whereas someone working indoors may go to the beach over the weekend with untanned skin and end up getting a sunburn.

Another controversial issue is the use of sun block. In recent decades there has been a big push for people to use sun block lotion but then there are others that say some of the chemicals used in sun block are not healthy either. However, there are some naturally based sun blocks that have recently become available. I think the best advice is to limit your exposure until your skin has adjusted and even then limiting exposure is a good idea. If you have fair skin that doesn't tan, obviously you're going to have to limit your skins exposure to the sun more than someone who tans easily. Tanning is your body's natural response and defense to protect the body against the damaging rays of the sun.

There have been many kinds of treatments for skin cancer. The most common is to surgically remove it. There is also cryosurgery, chemotherapy, immunotherapy, photodynamic therapy and radiation therapy which is also called radio therapy. There are also bio-oxidative and nutritional therapies which are natural alternative therapies.

One homeopathic alternative that I have heard of over the years is Bloodroot salve which comes from the Bloodroot plant (Sanguinaria Canadensis). It's a small flowering woodland plant found in different parts of the U.S and Canada that is also known by other names. It has been used by Native Americans historically for its curative properties. I have read many articles and reviews of individuals who have had good results removing skin abnormalities and spots of skin cancer using a quality Bloodroot salve product. One such product I've seen that has gotten a lot of good reviews is Frankin Thyme Bloodroot Skin Salve Sanguinaria Canadensis For Abnormal Skin. Generally, you cover the area to be treated with the salve and cover with a bandage for 24 hours. If abnormal cells are present, the herbs will continue to work for several days. It may take one or two treatments. Many people who have used it say it caused the abnormal tissue to scab over and then fall out, leaving healthy skin in its place and that it worked well. I have personally never used this type of product. Bloodroot has been used to treat various kinds of health problems as well. However, it is poisonous if taken internally in too large amount. If you are considering using a Bloodroot salve, I encourage you to do your own research on this subject including the different Bloodroot salve products that are available.

Another simple and inexpensive treatment I have heard of recently is topical iodine. Italian oncologist Dr. Tullio Simoncini says using topical iodine, such as what is available at local drug stores, is a very safe and effective treatment for skin cancer.

If you have a skin abnormality you should definitely have it looked at by a doctor to determine if it is skin cancer.

If you have skin cancer you should carefully consider all treatment options available.

I am against any chemotherapy because of its toxicity. I'm against radiation therapy because of the damage it does to healthy tissue. Ultimately, as with any kind of cancer, the underlying issue is the overall health of your body and your immune system. A healthy immune system that is operating properly will recognize and attack abnormal cells in the body. You can increase this effect by using potent nutritional products that stimulate the immune response such as vitamin C with bioflavonoids, selenium and vitamin D. Exercise and fresh air will help increase oxygen levels in your body tissues and sunlight will also help boost immune response. As with anything, it's important to have a healthy balance. Too much exercise or too much sun, for example, can have a negative effect also.

You are the patient and it's your body, do your own research, consider all of the options available and choose which treatment or treatments you believe are best.

CHAPTER 11

GENETICS AND CANCER

Recently there has been a lot of news coverage on the topic of genetic testing for the purpose of diagnosing a person's possible predisposition to developing cancer. The testing has to do with inherited genes that researchers believe may be related to the development of cancer. Famous people and average citizens have been in the news who have chosen to have mastectomy surgery because of a cancer diagnosis or simply because they tested positive for a gene that has been inherited from a parent who had cancer. Recently I listened to a radio broadcast on this subject where a healthy young woman in her 20s was planning to have a double mastectomy so she and her future children would not have to face it later in her life. It seems that a fear of cancer mindset has taken hold of our society. It's interesting to me that people spend their lives focused on the possibility or inevitability of getting cancer. That they are watching and waiting to receive the dreaded news from their doctor someday, yet they never invest any of that time and energy into researching and learning about the subject of cancer themselves first hand. It seems so many people have placed implicit trust in main stream medicine, assuming that the doctors they are dealing with possess all knowledge about cancer, and as if they are a nonprofit charitable organization whose sole purpose is to heal them with no interest in the profitability of what they do. No, hospitals, pharmaceutical companies and doctors are making a great deal of money in the cancer treatment industry. Every cancer patient is a very serious business prospect! One cancer patient can generate as much as $250,000. or more in income for the health care industry.

Doctors who do not buy into the idea of genetic predisposition say the argument against it is easy. Someone's mother and grandmother may have had breast cancer but what about their ancestors before them. Before the twentieth century cancer was a relatively rare disease. It's interesting to me that researchers who believe in the genetics argument never bring up the subject of other outside factors such as dietary habits, lifestyle and environmental factors. Woman are beginning to view their breasts as ticking time bombs, attached to their bodies, waiting to explode with cancer at some point in the future and kill them. (I'm not trying to be unkind in the things that I'm saying, rather I am making a point for those people who can benefit from this information at this time and in the future.)

When a doctor meets with a patient and discusses the issue of a family history of cancer, does he ever suggest the possibilities of other outside cancer causing factors? Here is the point; families hand down more than just genes to their children. They also pass on dietary habits, lifestyle habits and certain ways of thinking. All of these can contain things that can either work against or for the development of cancer. If a person really does have a genetic issue that predisposes them to disease more than others, that person's problem may be solved simply by giving greater attention to specialized nutrition. They may benefit from higher vitamin C and selenium intake and other nutrients as well.

In recent times other possible cancer causing factors have come to the forefront of discussion also, such as the effect of modern bras. It wasn't until the twentieth century that bra manufactures started using chemicals and synthetic materials including different kinds of rubber foam. There is now research that shows that some of these synthetic materials are out gassing chemical vapors, particularly when heated up to body temperature. Also some bra manufacturers have been found to be treating natural fabrics with harmful chemicals.

Another issue is that of constrained circulation due to the tightness of braziers. With impaired circulation, oxygen flow to the cells is reduced and toxins can, over time, become concentrated creating unhealthy, oxygen starved tissue. However, like anything else, there are some women whose bodies may never seem to be affected by synthetic materials or tight braziers, but then there are other people who will, because different individuals have varying physiological tolerances.

After all of the studies I've read on this subject it seems the healthiest breasts are ones that are not overly constrained by a bra and are not exposed to toxic chemicals. One study even claimed to show that breasts become firmer when they have to support their own weight. (This was from a French study that focused on women in their 20s and 30s.) Ultimately breast health is a whole body issue.

With all of the dietary, mental and environmental factors that people face today, is it any wonder why there are so many people developing disease. As I am describing in this book, an individual needs to take a whole person approach to the prevention and treatment of disease. There are many things a woman can do to prevent and cure breast cancer naturally and inexpensively without ever having to live life in fear. **If you take the time to learn about how a healthy body functions and the relationship between health, food and the environment, you can become a master of your own body and your own health!** You don't have to be afraid of cancer anymore!

CHAPTER 12

LEFT FOR DEAD

I had a neighbor a number of years ago that was diagnosed with bone cancer and sent home to die. She initially was under a doctor's care in regard to an unrelated surgical procedure she was scheduled to have. The doctor had all of her teeth pulled out to prepare her for the operation. (The doctors were concerned that bacteria might migrate from her teeth and gums to the point of surgery and cause infection.) Then the doctors diagnosed her with bone cancer so they canceled the surgery and sent her home to die with no hope.

This woman was a single mother with two small children living at home. I went to visit her when I heard about her condition. She looked like the picture of death and was sitting in her easy chair with the expectation that she would die of bone cancer. I felt sorry for the woman and told her I had some nutritional supplements that would help speed the healing of her gums. I said I also could give her some supplements to help her overcome cancer. I gave her the supplements with suggestions. I also gave her suggestions on healthy dietary and lifestyle changes. She was very interested in everything I had to say. I also prayed with her and gave her a little book called Gods Medicine, which is about divine healing.

The supplements I gave her were things I researched for myself and were natural and high potency. I gave her Vitamin C that came with citrus bioflavonoids, a shark cartilage supplement, sodium selenite, CoQ10 in a gel cap form, a multi vitamin, multi mineral, herbal supplement called Reliv Classic, that is well balanced and comes in a powder form, and a protein supplement. Six different products in all. I also gave her some healthy food as well. I gave her these things free of charge with dosage suggestions. I did not prescribe anything. She had no other options and was glad to try them.

In a short period of time, several months later, she was better and carrying on her normal life activities. She did not die from cancer, she became healthy and well again. What did I intend to accomplish through the supplements that I gave her? Three things, the supplements were intended to dramatically boost immune function, improve heart function and blood flow along with an increase in oxygen, and cause her body to become nutritionally balanced. Everything I gave her I had personally researched for myself. I had found clinical research studies that proved these supplements do specific things in the body. I also added the spiritual aspect because God can do things that cannot be done in the natural. I knew it would also give her peace in her heart and mind. This is the type of care medical doctors should be giving their patients in our health care system today. **There is no reason to leave any patient for dead that is still living!**

Here is one of the most important points I would like to make in this entire book. Both Dr. Lorrian Day and my neighbor were given up on by medical science. Dr. Day said in her initial efforts to treat her own cancer she wasn't doing certain things she needed to do and the cancer ended up spreading to the point that she became terminally ill. In her story she tells how she became so sick she could no longer hold food or water down. She was at home being cared for by her husband and came to the point where she was within hours of dying when she realized there were certain things she could do to sustain life. She asked her husband to take her to the hospital and asked the doctors to give her a hydration and nutritional enema. As her condition improved she said the Spirit of God began to reveal to her the simple dietary and lifestyle changes she needed to begin doing to reverse the cancer and regain her health. She said once she started doing those things it took 18 months for her body to make a complete recovery, naturally, without chemo, radiation or mutilating surgery. Here is what I believe; if a person is still alive and they begin doing the right things and stop doing the wrong things, cancer can be reversed! No one is without hope if they are still living!

Recently I saw a new ad for a certain cancer hospital where the question was asked, what is cancer? In the ad they described that cancer occurs when cells begin to replicate without the normal controls of the body. The cells can begin to interfere with vital functions and organs of the body. They went on to say that there are also different kinds of cancer cells that react differently to specific treatments. Although this particular cancer hospital offers alternative treatments that they seem to have had good success with, they echoed statements made by conventional medicine. **Conventional medicine says that cancer and cancer treatment is very complex! I could not disagree more strongly with that statement.** The best cancer doctor you could ever have, naturally speaking, is your own body! God created the body with a powerful healing capacity. The body is designed to fix itself. What you have to do is put the right nutrients in, along with the right care, and it will begin the process of repairing itself. When the body is biochemically balanced and healthy, the immune system will recognize cancer as an intruder and it will eliminate it, regardless of what kind of cancer it is or where it is. **This is cancer treatment made simple!** I believe the number one reason why conventional medicine makes cancer treatment seem so complex is because the pharmaceutical industry, hospitals and doctors want to be the ones dispensing the treatments. They want to control the industry because cancer treatment is big business and since there are so few people who understand their bodies and cancer, the cancer industry is able to perpetuate what they are doing!

CHAPTER 13

COLON CANCER: WHAT I WOULD DO IF I HAD IT

In my life time I have heard of and known many people who have been diagnosed with colon cancer and have received conventional cancer treatment for it, often including removal of part or all of the colon (large intestine.) People have colons for a purpose, it's needed to properly and fully digest the food that we eat. It also holds waste until a person is ready to eliminate. When a colon is removed it causes a lot of long term problems and complications. A person is limited in what and how they can eat and how much of the foods nutrients are absorbed by the body. It also means a person has to have a bag connected to their body for the rest of their life.

The reason why there is so much colon cancer in America is because many people eat a lot of processed, unhealthy, low fiber food on a regular basis. Here's how colon cancer forms. Let's say a person likes to eat fast food regularly and they like burgers, fries and soft drinks. These kinds of foods have virtually no fiber and eventually become difficult for the muscles of the digestive tract to move through the intestines. As a result of not enough fiber or water being present in their diet, they become constipated.

Bowel transit time can vary greatly depending on many different factors such as diet, activity level and medications being taken. According to a number of studies I looked at it can take between 24 and 72 hours for food to travel through the entire digestive system before being eliminated. However, I believe that a healthy person, who is eating the right amount of healthy foods and is getting the right amount of exercise, should actually have a bowel transit time less than 24 hours. It can even be as little as 7 to 12 hours depending on the food that has been eaten. For example, if you ingest a large amount of cayenne in your diet it can dramatically speed up bowel transit time. Normally, in a healthy person, a bowel movement should occur within an hour and half after a normal meal. (Also when you're getting enough fiber and water in your digestive tract, a bowel movement should only take a minute or two to eliminate). Conversely, a person eating the wrong foods, who is in a state of perpetual constipation, may take up to 3 days or more for their food to travel through the entire digestive system. During that time the unhealthy foods that have been eaten are rotting and putrefying in the intestines and the intestine walls are being exposed to this and absorbing it. The intestine walls eventually become irritated and toxified creating a cellular state of confusion in the colon tissue. This is how polyps, tumors and cancer start in the colon and other parts of the body. In addition, the high sugar soft drinks only help to fuel the growth of cancer cells. What is the solution? Instead of trying to poison, burn or cut out the sick tissue, we should simply reverse the harmful process that created the disease with the right foods, nutrients and lifestyle changes. Once again the best doctor you can choose for reversing disease (other than Jesus) is your own body. God created your body with a powerful ability to heal itself, you just add the right food, hydration, sleep, exercise and mental and spiritual state and your body will begin to heal wounds and eliminate cancer cells.

You can dramatically speed up this healing process by taking the right amount of nutritional supplements, which have proven potency, and have been clinically proven to speed healing and boost immune function. By taking the right dosages and combining or compounding different supplements that complement each other, a person can create a nuclear reaction of healing in the body! In other words, you're dealing with highly enriched or concentrated, highly potent nutrients. Tumors will shrink, wounds will heal, and cancer will disappear, all in a short period of time, with no negative side effects!

If I was diagnosed with colon cancer or any other kind of cancer or a tumor inside of my body, here is what I would do. I would begin eating a mostly vegan diet of whole foods such as fresh fruits, nuts and vegetables and whole grains foods. Some doctors recommend that some people avoid wheat or wheat gluten. It's up to you whether or not you want to include other grains in your diet. Some grains are healthier than others such as oats, which are lower than wheat on the glycemic index. I like to try different kinds of whole grain products like organic sprouted grain breads that do not contain flour. I also like to have whole grain Swiss muesli for breakfast from time to time. Swiss muesli is made up of pieces of dried fruit, nuts, seeds and different kinds of whole rolled, roasted grains. It's an excellent food for cleaning out the colon. However, with cancer most holistic experts say to focus mainly on a vegan diet and mostly vegetables that tend to have an alkaline effect in the body. If you do some research on this subject you will find a long list of fruits, nuts, vegetables and even some grains that fall into this category. Here is a partial list of vegetables: Carrots, celery, chard, cucumbers, bell peppers, broccoli, green beans, kale, leaks, lettuce, peas, rutabagas, spinach, and sprouts.

In regard to fruits and vegetables I would make a point to do some juicing to get more nutrients out of them. The NutriBullet brand juicer, for example, comes with a juicing book that has many different juicing combination ideas.

I would also eat all organic and Non-GMO (GMO stands for genetically modified organisms) if it was something I could afford to do. Non-GMO products are easy to find and usually not expensive. Organic food is generally more expensive than non-organic but definitely worth the extra cost. I would make sure I'm drinking enough water and I would only drink it purified or distilled so there is no chlorine or other contaminants in it. I would avoid all refined flour and sugar. I would abstain from artificial sweeteners like NutraSweet (aspartame) because of the negative health effects it has become associated with. I may eat some small amounts of animal protein but it would have to be free range and organic. Any dairy products would have to be unprocessed (no homogenization.) Until all cancer is gone I would limit animal protein to organic yogurt, and poached or soft boiled eggs.

By eating whole foods such as fruits, nuts, vegetables and whole grain foods along with drinking water throughout the day, I would get my bowel movements back to normal and create an environment in the intestines that will allow healing to begin.

I would begin taking a quality, balanced, multivitamin, mineral, herbal supplement to help get my body back into biochemical and nutritional balance. The best product that I have found is called Reliv Classic. It comes as a powder and is supposed to be mixed into water or juice. Then I would begin taking special supplements to speed the healing process like . . .

Vitamin C: I would take a quality vitamin C supplement that includes a healthy dose of bioflavonoids. I would take large doses, anywhere from 3.5 to 7 grams per day. One of the brands I'm currently using is Nature's Plus Super C Complex. Vitamin C is a water soluble vitamin that is not stored by the body, so any amount your body doesn't use is eliminated. Vitamin C can dramatically boost the immune response immediately and speed the healing of damaged tissues. It also increases the levels of hydrogen peroxide and oxygen in the blood. (When taking a new supplement always follow the dosage suggestion on the bottle to see how it affects your body before increasing to higher dosages.)

Selenium: I would also include a quality Selenium supplement like Sodium Selenite. Some experts say you can safely take up to 600 mcg per day. If you develop brittle hair or nails, skin rashes, nausea or garlic breath, these are signs you're getting too much. Some people have taken up to 6000 mcg per day for cancer therapy, however when you're compounding supplements you are going to get a synergistic effect and are probably better off testing smaller doses and then observing how its working in your body by how you feel and function. Begin with the suggested dosage.

Co Q10: I would also take a soft gel form of CoQ10 which gives energy to cell mitochondria. Smaller doses are good because it tends to build up in the body and it can cause your heart rate to increase if you're getting too much.

Shark Cartilage Powder: There have been many studies done on the health benefits of shark cartilage and one of the main things it has been found to do is shrink tumors. I would begin with the suggested dosage. Later I would consider increasing to 2, 750 mg capsules three times a day (6 capsules.)

Cayenne: Cayenne is considered the catalyst of all herbs. It is a powerful natural vasodilator and also gives energy to the whole body. In one study it was shown to have the ability to kill cancer cells in the prostate. I would begin by taking 1, 450 mg capsule containing 40,000 heating units, with a meal. It could create discomfort if a person has polyps or cancer in the colon but if it doesn't cause too much discomfort it will improve circulation and speed the healing process. It has even been used to help heal stomach ulcers. Eventually I would take 1 with each meal to aid healing (2 or 3 capsules per day). Sometimes cayenne will cause my heart rate to speed up. I found I can control this by taking 1, 450 mg Valerian root capsule for every Cayenne capsule I take. You have to see what works best for you.

Probiotic: I would take a quality probiotic supplement to make sure there is enough of the right kind of bacteria in the colon for healthy digestion.

Protein Supplement: The body needs a healthy, quality source of protein every day to repair and maintain itself. Organic rice protein is a great way to add extra protein to your diet. If you make it into a protein drink you can take it with you and take some of it in-between meals wherever you are. I usually will carry a small personal cooler in the car with me that's just large enough for some healthy food items, a protein drink and some water. If you're on an all vegan diet this can really help you get enough high quality protein in your daily diet. Personally, I like to mix whey isolate, egg white and rice protein powders together to create a mixture that is more digestible and palatable. I mix measured amounts of all three protein powders together with a 50/50 mix of water and milk in a blender or shaker container. You can add fruit, vegetables or natural flavor as well.

When taking a new supplement it's a good idea to begin with a small amount to see if you have any kind of adverse reaction to it and to see how it individually affects your body. If you're taking a fat soluble vitamin, like vitamin E, it's important to realize that fat soluble vitamins are stored by the body and therefore you can get too much. If while taking supplements you begin to feel sluggish or toxic, it may be time to cut back or take a break from taking those supplements and let your body use what's currently in your body. Most supplements are recommended to be taken with food. The number one supplement that is recommended to be taken on an empty stomach is Arginine.

Rest: Getting to bed at 9 or 10 pm at the latest is necessary for aligning your sleeping hours with your internal biological clock. Sleep is the time when our bodies rest, repair and heal. You should get 7 to 8 hours of sleep every night. Not getting enough or having erratic sleeping habits can actually lead to the development of disease. Your biological clock aligns itself with daylight and dark due to hormones that are released by the body in the presence of light and darkness. Also make sure you allow sufficient time for food from your last meal to digest before going to bed. Allow at least three hours after a full meal before you sleep unless the meal is a very light meal comprised of easy to digest food. Allow one hour after a protein drink.

Work: There are some experts, like Dr. Day, that recommend taking time off of work until you have made a complete recovery from cancer, so you can give your full attention and energy to getting well.

Exercise: Walking outside in the fresh air and sunshine is ideal. Walking is a low impact, low stress exercise that gets the blood flowing and increases oxygen levels throughout the body. You can even create endorphin production through walking. When a person is ill and trying to overcome disease, it's important to also get fresh air to stimulate healing and the immune system. Indoor air often contains a certain amount of air pollution unless you have a really good air purifier.

Sunshine: Having exposure to sunshine gives the body a chance to produce its own vitamin D naturally, which is critical to health and immune function. If I couldn't get enough sun exposure because of living in a cold northern climate, I would go to a tanning salon several times a week to make up for the lack of sunlight. Having a limited, balanced exposure to the sun or tanning bed lights has been proven to have certain positive health effects, including fighting depression. Negative health effects can arise when a person has too much exposure to UV radiation, like someone who tans every day, so once again the key is maintaining a healthy balance of exposure. In the winter I generally tan twice a week. I make a point not to allow any burning to occur.

Spirituality: Since God made our bodies it would make sense to take time to seek God in prayer and in scripture reading daily. Attending to this first thing every morning is the best way to do it, by giving God first place. The Bible has a lot to say about healing and the things we should do to put ourselves in a position for healing and answered prayer. Having an attitude of forgiveness and thankfulness are also vitally important to healing, answered prayer and knowing God. There are a lot of good scriptural Bible based books available on the subject of divine healing. In this book I share some scriptures on the subject.

CHAPTER 14

BIO-OXIDATIVE THERAPIES AND OTHER NATURAL CURES

A person doesn't have to look very hard to find information on natural therapies that have been approved and used in other countries for decades but continue to be rejected or sidelined by main stream medicine here in the U.S. Ozone therapy is among them. Bio-oxidative therapies refer to the therapeutic use of oxygen, medical ozone and hydrogen peroxide. All occur naturally in nature. **Ozone is not air pollution** but is a normal part of our environment. Although ozone may form in smog due to the ultraviolet radiation from the sun on air pollutants, ozone is best known as the fresh air smell after an electrical storm. Ozone is a short lived gas that is created when oxygen has been subjected to electrical current or sufficient ultraviolet light. It then begins reverting back to oxygen. Hydrogen peroxide or H2O2 forms in rain water as rain drops fall through ozone. Ozone is O3 while oxygen is O2. Ozone and hydrogen peroxide are two of nature's greatest cleaning agents. Ozone may irritate the lungs if breathed in too high of a concentration for too long, but when used properly it can have a powerful healing effect in the body. Ozone therapy focuses on the absorption of ozone through the skin rather than breathing it. There is also (DIV) Direct Intravenous Ozone Gas administration.

Ozone has been used to purify water and treat patients for more than 160 years. Ozone therapy was accepted medicine in the U.S beginning around 1870 until 1933. In the 1930's, shortly after the Food and Drug Administration became known by its current name, it banned its use. Countries such as Germany, Russia, and Cuba have been using ozone therapy with great success for decades. In Germany ozone therapy was used in the 1930's and has been used in main stream medicine there since the 1950's. It has been estimated that more than ten thousand German doctors have used ozone therapy, on millions of patients, for many different diseases, and with a high rate of success. Ozone becomes hydrogen peroxide, in part, when it enters the blood. It has a super oxygenating and cleansing effect in the body without the toxic side effects so commonly associated with pharmaceutical drugs. Generally, it has a powerful rejuvenating effect on organs and body tissues and speeds the healing process. It also helps to modulate or bring about correct immune function.

Ozonation also safely and effectively kills pathogens in the blood including HIV! Ozone and hydrogen peroxide give off free radical oxygen atoms. The thin cell walls of viral and bacterial infections have no defense against these high energy atoms and are ripped open as a result. Human cell walls are thicker and are more resistant to this oxygenating free radical process. Ozone therapy has been effective in treating HIV, cancer, heart disease, arthritis, diabetes and many other diseases.

Ozone and hydrogen peroxide are inexpensive and can be self-administered through various means. Hydrogen peroxide therapy has even been used to cure emphysema. It does this by dissolving plaque that has built up on the lung alveoli as the hydrogen peroxide enters the lung tissue from the blood stream. Hydrogen peroxide is produced naturally by our white blood cells but supplementing is useful when the body is not producing enough to overcome disease. **Bio-oxidative therapy is probably the greatest scientific discovery of modern medicine because of its safety, effectiveness, versatility and low cost.**

In May of 1982 the Sixth World Ozone Conference was held in Washington D.C. During this conference many medical papers were reviewed on the successes of world recognized specialists of the treatment of many different diseases. Presently there are twenty-four countries that allow the use of ozone therapy. There are also 14 U.S states that now allow doctors to use it without fear of persecution. According to the American Academy of ozonotherapy there are professional medical ozone therapy societies in over ten countries worldwide. To the best of my knowledge the FDA has not yet given full approval for ozone therapy. However medical doctors who are participating in ozone research may use it under an Institutional Review Board (IRB). All data collected must be forwarded to the FDA for analysis. In other words, the FDA is still investigating the safety and effectiveness of ozone even though it's been used and proven safe and effective in other countries for many decades.

My Personal Experiences with Ozone

In the last 20 years I have purchased a number of different kinds of air purifiers to improve the quality of the air in my bedroom and other living spaces. Last year I bought a popular brand that has a cleanable HEPA filter and also draws the air past an ultraviolet light and electrically charged ionizer. I bought one and liked it so much I bought three more for about one hundred dollars each. They're advertised as air purifiers but also produce varying amounts of ozone depending on the fan speed setting. There are a lot of air purifiers that come with ionizers that produce varying amounts of ozone. On mine, finding the right fan speed setting creates an optimal mix of O2 and O3 in the air. Too much ozone can have negative effects and can be irritating but having the right amount gives a sense that there is much more available oxygen in the air. Having the right amount of ozone in a room is also very invigorating. Even though the oxygen in the room is the same, the creation of O3 or ozone creates more individual free radical oxygen atoms in the air as the ozone begins to break down. It's my theory that the individual oxygen atoms are absorbed through the skin faster than the larger molecules. At any rate the presence of ozone in the air makes the oxygen in the air more available for use by the body. In my experiences, depending on the fan setting, it can seem like there is twice as much available oxygen in the room. Just make sure you are not irritating your lungs with too much O3. Sometimes I shut mine off for a while to allow the air to normalize in the room again. I have found that my air purifiers have been extremely effective at removing odors and air pollution from the rooms they are in. The effectiveness of removing odors is largely due to the oxidizing effect of ozone on surfaces that can harbor odors. Waking up in the morning with my air purifier cleaning the air is like waking up to breathing fresh mountain air. Once again, if you have a purifier that produces ozone, make sure the settings are correct so you are not getting too much. Generally, too much ozone in the air will be irritating and can cause your chest and lungs to feel heavy.

There are more and more books and websites coming out on this subject including ones that give specific directions and protocols on how to treat yourself with bio-oxidative therapies such as using food grade hydrogen peroxide orally. Sometimes when you buy the food grade hydrogen peroxide it will come with instructions on its many uses. Hydrogen peroxide is like ozone but in a liquid form. There are also many kinds of ozone generators available today. If you desire to find an experienced health care professional to provide you with bio-oxidative therapy I would do an internet search for sites that provide lists of these licensed and experienced professionals. Take time to do background checks and check customer referrals.

CHAPTER 15

HEART HEALTH

Another amazing natural cure is cayenne as a standardized supplement. I mentioned it previously but I will say more about it here in regard to heart health. Cayenne is said to be the catalyst of all other herbs. Cayenne upon ingestion immediately dilates the vascular system increasing oxygen and lowering blood pressure, thus making it easier for the heart to function. It stimulates and gives energy to the heart and the entire body. It is so powerful it has been used effectively to stop heart attacks from both blockages and stress. It can also immediately open a blockage from a stroke. (Stroke is the number one cause of disability for people over the age of 50.) Cayenne is a natural food substance that rejuvenates and feeds cardiac and other tissues in the body. Taken regularly cayenne also has a cleansing effect on the vascular system, cleaning plaque from the artery walls. Cayenne stimulates the immune system and healing throughout the body. Cayenne has been used for ages for medicinal purposes for many different health issues.

Cayenne is low cost and when taken orally in capsule form has no negative side effects except feeling some internal warmth from it. It's best taken with food when possible. When I take cayenne and I haven't had any food to eat beforehand, I usually will take one valerian root capsule for each cayenne capsule. Just as cayenne can instantly stimulate the heart, valerian can almost instantly calm heart function. Cayenne can cause the heart to speed up but valerian will counteract this effect. Here are the names of some other heart supplements I have used. CoQ10 or ubiquinol, which gives energy to cell mitochondria. L-arginine (an amino acid which dilates the vascular system and produces nitric oxide in the blood, which is necessary for muscle recovery after exercise). Alfalfa tablets, vitamin C with bioflavonoids (which can clean and strengthen blood vessels), omega-3 fish oil and quercetin which is a super antioxidant. I suggest when taking any supplements, you read the label and check for the possibility of negative interactions with anything else you're taking. Naturally, if you're taking prescription drugs you want to pass it by your health care provider and check for the possibility of negative interactions. Some doctors are open to natural supplements and some see them as unwanted competition. When taking supplements you should begin with small amounts until you know how it affects your body. Be careful not to take arginine and cayenne together because you can get an over vasodilation which can be very alarming! I have found that after I had become accustomed to both separately, I could take both at the same time in small amounts, however I normally take them separately and I think this is best. The couple of times where I have taken too much, I would dilute it by drinking water or milk and eating some food.

  There are a lot of heart medications on the market today. One of the most popular are statin drugs. Statin drugs control the amount of cholesterol produced by the liver but with many potentially harmful side effects. If I was a cardiologist that knew the risks involved in taking such drugs, I would not consider prescribing them. It wouldn't be in the patient's best interest considering all of the safe and highly effective natural alternatives that work with the body rather than against it. Statin drugs have been linked to many serious side effects such as memory loss, muscle pain, liver injury, cancer, diabetes and even death!

There are now many doctors who believe high cholesterol levels are not even the real issue in the area of heart disease but that the main problem is diet. The body produces cholesterol for a purpose, to coat and protect muscle tissue and organs. If you don't have enough, your muscle tissue can begin to break down quickly. Studies of the inside of veins, arteries and the heart show that eating foods that contain refined and or molecularly altered ingredients can scrape and scour their inner walls. Once these walls are damaged they try to heal themselves and food substances can begin to build up on these scab spots eventually creating a blockage that can result in a heart attack or stroke. Refined flour, sugar, homogenized dairy products, hydrogenated vegetable oils and fats and oils high in omega 6 fatty acids are believed to be the main culprits in causing damage to the cardiovascular system, among causing other health problems as well. I'm sure a person can eat small amounts of these things from time to time without causing damage, but the problem is there are a lot of people who are eating too many of these things every day and they are taking a toll on their health. Also animal fat from stall fed animals is believed to be another culprit because the chemistry of the fat is unhealthy and different from free range animals eating their natural diet of grass. People are getting too many omega 6 fatty acids from grain fed animals and fried foods and not enough omega 3 fatty acids which are found in grass fed animal protein and certain kinds of fish, such as wild salmon.

In addition to diet being a significant part of the equation in heart disease, there are also other factors that can play a role such as toxins in our environment. Some experts have even pointed to the detrimental effect of mercury on the cardiovascular system, which can come from Amalgam dental fillings that are in your own mouth. In my case the thing that affected my heart health the most were pollutants in the air in my own home.

For the majority of my life I never had any problems with my heart. As a young person I could play any sport and never experienced any health problems. I can thank my Mother for making our family aware of healthy food choices when I was in grade school. As a young person, in my teens, I got involved in weight lifting and bodybuilding. After a while I built up my body, increased my body weight and began lifting some pretty heavy weights. As a junior in high school I weighed about 165 pounds at about 6 ft. After high school graduation I had worked up to 175 pounds mainly through my weight lifting program. Then, over the next few years I became very focused on increasing muscle mass through weightlifting and by my early 20s had gotten up to 253 pounds. My best lift was doing corner rowing by putting one end of an Olympic bar in a corner and putting 45 pound plates on the other end. The exercise is for the back. Bending over I would straddle the bar at the weighted end, with my back toward the corner. I would grip the bar in one place with both hands, behind the weights, and pull it toward me in a rowing motion. I got up to lifting ten 45 pound plates for 8 repetitions. That's nearly 500 pounds. That's a lot of work for the heart! Sometimes I worked out so hard I would feel sick to my stomach after the workout but never had the slightest trouble with my heart or lungs.

In 2006 I bought a house in the city of Marinette that was built in 1970. It was a foreclosure that had sat empty for more than two years. It was an unusual home, a one of a kind custom built home in an exclusive part of the city. The house was 4800 square feet with vaulted ceilings and exposed beams in the second level. The price had been marked down so much I decided to buy it as investment and to initially live in it as well.

When I walked into the house for the first time I knew there were strong chemical odors in the air. I thought this occurred because the house had been closed up for 2 ½ years. I figured the odor problem could be solved without too much trouble. Maybe just opening all the windows and airing it out would do it. However, after living in the house for several years I realized the problem was much more serious. To make a long story short, I concluded the chemical odors were coming from the particle board sub floor, the carpeting and all the cleaning chemicals left in the carpeting over the many years it had been cleaned.

After several years of living in this house I began to feel sick. I realized the house had a serious problem with VOCs (volatile organic chemicals) in the air. On January 2nd of 2008 I decided to remove all of the carpeting in the master bedroom. That night, actually early the next morning, I went to the emergency room because I was having trouble breathing. My bronchial passages had become constricted. I had a reaction to the allergens that were worked up when I tore out the carpeting combined with VOCs that were already in the air. The doctors in the emergency room began asking me some odd questions about what I had been doing. Apparently they thought I may have inhaled something on purpose. Finally, they put me on an inhaler that contained a mist that opened up my bronchial passages. Before I left they gave me some antihistamine tablets and said I should take them if it happens again. The bill for my brief visit was $800!

After this event I began sleeping at the caretaker's apartment at the youth center I operate, where there were no VOCs in the air. It had natural wood flooring. If I felt better I would stay at the house and open the windows in the room where I was staying. So, as a result, I was not totally free from exposure to the VOCs in the house in Marinette. Then later that year, in the late summer, I drove to the Milwaukee area for work and went to a grocery store to pick up a few things. Suddenly I felt something wrong in my throat. Like something was tightening up. Then my heart beat began to speed up noticeably. I realized something was seriously wrong with my heart. I went back to the house where I stay when I'm working in that area and laid down and began to breathe heavily to try to take in more oxygen. I could feel my heart beat was much faster than normal and also weaker or shallower. I probably should have gone to the hospital but I decided not to. If I had gone to the hospital, doctors could have possibly brought it under control right away. I'm not really sure. However, the next day I remembered some things I read in a book about herbs and decided to try what I had read. I went to a health food store and bought some cayenne capsules and some valerian root capsules. The cayenne seemed to take stress off my heart and lungs and the valerian root slowed my heart rate down back to normal. I found some supplements that gave me immediate relief and seemed to have solved my problem. However, through the coming days, weeks and months I realized that something was seriously wrong with my heart. My heart had become weaker and much more unstable. I concluded that the VOCs that I had been exposed to for years, in the house I had bought in Marinette, had built up in my body tissues, my heart and my lungs. Over the next few years I experienced numerous stress heart attacks where I sometimes felt I might experience total heart failure. Generally, the attacks would occur if I exercised too much or if I didn't get enough sleep or a combination of both. Anything that seemed to create too much stress could bring about the onset of a stress heart attack.

When I felt an attack coming I would begin to feel uneasy as I felt tension begin to build in my chest area. The symptoms I experienced during an actual attack would be tightness in the neck, sweatiness, significant pain in my heart, weakness in the legs, and a sense that my heart was struggling with every beat. However, I discovered that taking several cayenne capsules (450 mg capsules containing 40,000 heating units each) could stop the stress heart attack within a few minutes. In some cases, I have taken as many as 5 at a time. Then an hour later I would literally feel like a new man because of the energy that the cayenne had released into my body tissues.

Then after I had been using cayenne for a while I read an article about bodybuilders using a combination of free form amino acids before sleep to help rebuild muscle during the night. The combination was arginine, (also known as L-arginine) and ornithine. I decided to try it and found that it also seemed to help the recovery of my heart. I began using L-arginine- ornithine with L-glutamine, taurine and creatine. I found using this combination of amino acids was more effective than using cayenne, but also different. I found that my heart function became noticeably stronger and stable after using the arginine-ornithine combination. It also helped the recovery of other injured muscles. Several years later I found out that NO, (nitric oxide) which is produced from arginine in the body, had been the subject of thousands of medical research studies and it was found to aid in the recovery of many different health problems. It relaxes blood vessels, keeps them smooth and has even been shown to reverse CVD (cardiovascular disease). Nitric oxide is also considered to be the most powerful natural antioxidant produced in the body. In 1998 the Nobel Prize was awarded to a group of researchers for the discovery of nitric oxide as a signaling molecule in the cardiovascular system. The effect of arginine in the vascular system has been shown to be so powerful that some doctors who use to prescribe statin drugs have replaced statins with arginine to get a much better overall health effect and without any of the negative side effects associated with statin drugs. I read about one cardiologist that stopped referring patients to heart surgeons for heart bypass surgery and angioplasty because of his discovery of arginine.

In addition to using these supplements in the recovery of my heart I also used moderate exercise and made sure I was getting sufficient sleep, all of which are key factors in recovery. I found that walking on a treadmill or outside at a moderate pace, anywhere from a 16 to 18 minute mile pace, for a minimum of 1 mile, three times a week, had a very noticeable positive effect on regulating heart function. In short, I noticed my heart function was becoming stronger and much more normal from the regular walking. Eventual my heart improved to the point that I could begin doing some running with the walking. Since my main interest is weight lifting, in regard to exercise, I don't put a lot of emphasis on running.

Eight years later my heart has vastly improved to the point that I can lift heavy weights again and even swing a 20 pound sledge hammer. I would not say that my heart has recovered 100% but I believe it is continually improving as long as I continue to do the right things and make a point to not over stress it. In August of 2013 I posted a series of three You Tube videos titled "Breaking Concrete the old fashioned way" where I'm breaking the concrete top of a well pit with a 20 pound sledge hammer. I demolished the entire thing myself and my heart was able to handle the workout.

Something I recently discovered is that if I need a pick me up, like an energy drink or coffee, I have come to the conclusion that caffeine is not ideal in regard to heart health and I have decided to either take cayenne or amino acids when I'm feeling drowsy and need to stay alert. Recently, when I wasn't feeling particularly well, I had to drive a long distance to a job site. I decided to take cayenne and valerian root capsules throughout the day to stay alert and help heart function at the same time. I would take one of each at the same time, every few hours (usually with food in my stomach). At the end of the day I may have taken a total of 5 or 6 of each. Instead of feeling wired like you would from caffeine I felt refreshed and well with no negative side effects! The outcome was very positive and lasting.

Clearly there are a lot of people out there who enjoy caffeinated beverages like coffee and energy drinks. You have to decide what works best for you. The main difference between caffeine and cayenne is that cayenne nourishes the body with real energy and nutrients while caffeine acts as a temporary stimulant that does not provide any actual energy or nutritional benefit. There are some energy drinks that contain caffeine from natural sources such as organic green coffee beans or contain other naturally sourced stimulants. It seems these are less likely to cause a person to feel over stimulated or wired afterword.

My final word on heart health is that if you want to maintain a healthy heart or even reverse heart disease, regardless of age, it can be achieved through maintaining consistency in healthy lifestyle and dietary practices. It's important to engage in regular exercise. It's important to consume healthy whole foods and avoid processed foods including foods that have a lot of added sugar, salt and unhealthy oils and fats. To get enough quality sleep and reduce stress levels. To avoid toxins that can build up in body tissues and affect the heart and to use the latest supplements available to increase cardiovascular health.

As a recap, my top 5 favorite heart supplements are cayenne, arginine, CoQ10, valerian and alfalfa tablets. All of these supplements do something different. Some give instantly noticeable results while some others take time to cause a noticeable effect. Cayenne, arginine and valerian all give immediate results while CoQ10 and alfalfa take time to give noticeable results. Right now I am taking 2, 100 mg gel caps of CoQ10 per day from a company called Natural Factors. I'm also taking 8 to 10 alfalfa tablets from Shaklee. Both of these supplements have given noticeable results. The CoQ10 gradually replenishes the heart, and cells throughout the body, when the body's natural production and supply of

CoQ10 have been diminished. Lowered levels of CoQ10 can occur from stress, toxins and aging. Alfalfa provides magnesium and other nutrients which support calm and consistent heart function.

Because of the latest knowledge about cardiovascular health in regard to diet, exercise, nutritional supplements and new non-invasive therapies such as EECP, it's my opinion, and that of many experts, that certain current conventional methods of dealing with heart disease have become outdated. Heart bypass surgery, stints, angioplasty and the use of statin drugs and blood thinners should be retired for these better, safer more economical solutions.

CHAPTER 16

REPLACE OR REJUVENATE?

Joint replacement and organ replacement are becoming more common in our modern times. However, the living tissues in the body that make up our organs are designed to repair themselves and the cells the tissues are made of are designed to replace themselves. The main reasons why organs and joints wear out before their time is due to dietary and lifestyle reasons. Look at the way people care for their bodies and the things they eat, is it any wonder? We work hard, we play hard. We abuse our bodies and then burn the candle at both ends, not getting enough sleep, the time during which the body repairs itself. Many people drink everything but pure water, while eating dead processed foods full of additives and chemicals. Then they smoke cigarettes, drink liquor, take drugs. All of these chemicals have to be processed by the organs of our bodies and then filtered out so they can be excreted because they don't belong. After the body has been going through this vicious cycle for years, something has to give.

The answer to a body that is wearing out is not a complicated issue. Simply reverse the dietary and lifestyle trends that caused the problems. Begin by detoxifying the body while properly nourishing it. Once again start eating healthy, unprocessed whole foods, like fresh fruits, nuts, vegetables and whole grains. Ideally you want things that haven't been corrupted with chemical pesticides and fertilizers, so buy organic when you can. Also start drinking purified water as your beverage of choice, such as distilled or reverse osmosis. Then you need to begin getting to bed at a reasonable hour in order to get enough sleep. You may even need to take a nap at some point in the day. If you are looking to recover from a worn out joint or organ, getting sufficient rest is a critical key in recovery.

The next point in rejuvenating a joint or an organ is taking special supplements that will speed the recovery process. For example, if you are looking to rebuild the cartilage in a worn out joint, start taking a quality glucosamine chondroitin supplement. There are many other natural herbs and supplements available that can be taken for joint health, along with glucosamine chondroitin for maximum effect. I also take Reliv Classic along with alfalfa tablets. Reliv also makes a product called Arthaffect. There are many other natural nutritional products available out there that are formulated to rebuild and restore healthy joint function. When you compound products that complement each other, you can get a very effective synergistic effect in a short period of time. You may notice a difference in a few days or it may take a couple of weeks to a month.

If I had a weak heart or problems with other organs, some of the main supplements that I would first look at using would be arginine, cayenne, CoQ10 or ubiquinol, alfalfa and selenium for example. You also need a balance of all necessary nutrients. In addition to nutritional therapy, bio-oxidative therapies such as ozone therapy have also had great success in this area. It has been shown to be low cost and very effective.

Finally, it's important to get the right kind of exercise on a regular basis. Proper exercise is a necessary key to healing and recovery. Regular exercise is a necessary key to maintaining proper healthy heart function and oxygen levels in the body. Normal healthy hormone levels are also maintained through regular exercise.

Through all of the studies that I have looked at and through my own personal experiences, I believe any living tissue in the body can be rejuvenated through these methods. Some tissues are designed to recover faster while others may take a longer period of time. However, I believe no matter what the problem is, once a person starts doing the right things, noticeable improvement should come about in a relatively short period of time.

Usually people begin noticing these kind of health problems as they age. Clearly our bodies do not recover as fast as they did at a younger age. It's logical that as the body ages your nutritional needs will increase and you are going to have to give more attention to properly taking care of the body in order to enjoy normal, healthy use and function.

CHAPTER 17

MENTAL HEALTH

Mental health, just like physical health, comes from maintaining balance in life. We see in the scriptures that we are more than just a physical body living in a physical world. We are spirit, soul and body. We are spiritual beings created in the image and likeness of God. We have a mind along with emotions and we live in a physical body. Here is a passage of scripture that reveals this fact.

And the very God of peace sanctify you wholly; and I pray God your whole spirit and soul and body be preserved blameless unto the coming of our Lord Jesus Christ. I Thessalonians 5:23

In order to maintain good mental health you must care for all of these areas in your life. However, the same is really true for physical health as well because all three of these areas are interconnected. If you're not taking care of your spiritual health and mental health, your body is going to suffer.

From the physical standpoint your brain and your body are like complex chemistry sets that need to be kept in balance in order to be healthy. If you're not eating right, sleeping right or getting proper exercise, it's going to affect your overall chemistry balance and it's going to affect your mental health to one degree or another. How you care for your overall health has a direct connection to your overall sense of wellbeing.

We also need healthy social interaction and healthy relationships with other people because that is how we are designed. We should seek to be around people who are positive, who are encouraging and supportive. We should seek to spend time around people who are going in the right direction and doing what is necessary to succeed in life.

Another important point about mental health, in regard to relating to others, is take time to take your eyes off of your own needs and look to what you can do to help others less fortunate than yourself. Take time to reach out to others and be a giver. What can you do to help others? What can you do to serve God? Take time to find out what your calling in life is to help others and make the world a better place.

The liberal soul shall be made fat: and he that watereth shall be watered also himself. Proverbs 11:25

First and foremost, we are spiritual beings and we have spiritual requirements that we need to attend to or we will never truly be happy, fulfilled or healthy. Take time to seek God in your life and read his word.

My son, attend to my words; incline thine ear unto my sayings. Let them not depart from thine eyes; keep them in the midst of thine heart. For they are life unto those that find them, and health to all their flesh. Proverbs 4:20-22

We need prayer in our lives. Take time to pray, take time for self-examination, take time to repent of any sins you may have committed, take time to forgive. Take time to pray for your enemies, that God would help them and intervene in their lives (Matthew 5:43-48). You can even pray that God would give you favor with your enemies. Take time to get right with God.

We need to gather together as a body of believers for church. Church should be the corner stone of our society because it's there that we join together with an attitude of faith, hope and love, to worship God, to hear the word of God (which tells us how we should live) and to fellowship with one another.

Real mental health is comprised of maintaining a balance of all of these things. God created each part of our being, spirit, soul and body. Happiness and mental health are things we should give thanks for as gifts from God. We should endeavor to live in harmony with God and our fellow man, our brother and our sister and it is then that we can experience wellbeing in the area of mental health.

CHAPTER 18

PHARMACUETICAL HELL AND THE ELDERLY

One of the greatest challenges facing our nation today is the financial burden of our growing elderly population. Our nation is faced with the stark reality of the increasing health care costs, nursing home costs and drug costs of the elderly. I have worked in nursing home ministry for 20 years and have observed the plight of the elderly in terms of health care. I have seen them in their wheel chairs, suffering with arthritis, Alzheimer's, dementia and many other serious health issues. I've heard their cries for help and even their screams from their rooms. I've seen the numerous drugs they have to take every day. I also had a very graphic dream once about this topic. In the dream I was walking down the hallway of a nursing home I have been to numerous times. As I was walking I looked into one of the open doorways to see an elderly woman I knew and saw a very disturbing scene. I saw she was bent in half and sealed in a plastic bag stewing in her own bodily fluids. The dream was so unusual and so real I knew it was a dream with an important meaning. What the plastic bag represents are sedation drugs that are secretly given to patients that are acting up and are given when a nurse feels this is the easiest way to deal with problematic disturbances even though there may be some other real health issues involved. I know about this practice because it was the subject of a television expose' on little known practices of nursing homes that I saw a number of years ago. It is known as chemical restraint and is used as a form of behavioral management even though it can lead to injury and death. This is not so much a criticism of the nursing homes I have been to but perhaps more a criticism of the status quo of our health care system in general.

I believe the health of our elder population could be dramatically improved if our health care system would get up to speed with what other countries are doing. Ozone whirlpool therapy and cutting edge nutritional therapy, along with healthy dietary changes would be a great place to start. Water aerobics and therapy would also be very valuable. The problem that I have noticed is that most nursing homes put a lot of emphasis on prescribing drugs. When it comes to nutrition, the foods that are served are often average institutional foods that are generally low in nutritional value. Most nursing homes are a long way away from optimal health care. In fact, most nursing homes are actually helping their residents become more dependent on health care whether they know it or not. I believe the bottom line is a combination of concerns about cost along with a lack of knowledge and innovation. The influence of the pharmaceutical industry also plays a large part since doctors are the ones prescribing the drugs.

When people age, their nutritional needs increase dramatically. What the elderly need is increased customized nutrition which should include whole organic foods. They should also have a certain amount of regular exposure to fresh air and sunshine for natural production of serotonin, vitamin D and general wellness. In regard to physical therapy, they should all be required to engage in walking or aquatic exercises on a regular basis as an example.

With the right changes in health care, the elderly could be more independent, more productive and enjoy a much better quality of life. It is my belief that the burden on our health care system could be greatly reduced!

CHAPTER 19

"AIDS HAS ITS PLACE IN THE WORLD NO MORE"

On 10/19/2011 I heard the Spirit of God say, "AIDS has its place in the world no more." God has the cure for AIDS in the natural and the supernatural.

A person could look at this word in several different ways. In recent times nations who have had the worst problems with HIV/AIDS have had success controlling the spread of the disease and treating it. There has been a lot of effort put towards the control and treatment of the disease by other nations and charitable organizations which is all very good news. However, rarely do you ever hear about treating the disease without drugs or hear about an actual cure for HIV/AIDS, which is what I would like to discuss in this chapter.

Several years ago I looked up the website of the world famous Mayo Clinic in Rochester Minnesota. I was reviewing the information on their HIV/AIDS page. It began by saying . . .

"There is no cure for HIV/AIDS, but a variety of drugs can be used in combination to control the virus."

There was also a section entitled "Treatment Can Be Difficult" where some of the drug side effects were listed such as . . .

Nausea, vomiting or diarrhea

Abnormal heartbeats

Shortness of breath

Skin rash

Weakened bones

Bone death, particularly in the hip joints

How is it possible that in this day, that supposedly some of the world's most intelligent doctors could not know about all of the studies that have shown that there is a way to safely deactivate (or kill) the HIV virus both in and out of the body. How is it these doctors are not aware of what is going on in other countries that are apparently more advanced in medicine and health care than we are? Or could it be these doctors are also part of the Great American Health Care Cover Up?

Previously I have already spoken of treatments that touch on the subject of HIV/AIDS. Ozone therapy has been successfully used to eliminate the HIV virus in the body and in blood taken out of the body as well. It is a normal and accepted treatment in counties that have legalized bio-oxidative therapies, and has been used for decades. There have been many studies done on the effectiveness of ozone to kill bacterial, viral and fungal infections safely.

In 1992 there was a major study done in Canada, overseen by the Surgeon General of the Canadian Armed Forces, that showed ozonating blood used for transfusion was 100 percent effective in deactivating (killing) the HIV virus. **It is particularly interesting to note that such a highly esteemed landmark study, done by our Canadian neighbors on blood supply purification, was never given any serious publicity by our medical establishment here in the U.S. This single official Canadian study alone is enough to show that there is something seriously and fundamentally wrong with our health care system in America.** There have been studies done in the U.S, Russia and Germany. The first known successful clinical studies on HIV/AIDS patients was done in Germany in the early to mid-1980's. I have found that there are many websites on the internet that are providing more and more information on this subject. From listing the many studies that have been done, to how therapies are administered, to clinics that now offer these therapies. Here are some website resources on this subject:

Family Health News

Natural News

Mercola.com

Dr. Robert Rowen's website

American Academy of Ozontherapy.

www.whale.to/v/mccabe.html,

www.oxygenhealingtherapies.com/ozone_oxygen_therapies.html
and countless more.

Also for at least 20 years it has been known that selenium is a key nutrient needed in the treatment of AIDS. Dr. Will Taylor first reported on the subject of AIDS and selenium depletion in the Journal of Medicinal Chemistry in August 1994. It is now known that the primary cause of the development of AIDS is selenium depletion which also leads to lowered levels of the antioxidant glutathione, which is produced by the body. Studies have shown that individuals who maintain the highest levels glutathione remain the healthiest and live the longest. **Here is a critical key about HIV/AIDS.** When a person becomes infected with the HIV virus and the virus begins to replicate and spread in the body, it searches out and robs the body of selenium, which is essential to proper immune function. The nation of Senegal Africa has the lowest level of AIDS of all African nations, at 1.77 percent and also has selenium rich soil. Senegal also has one of the lowest rates of cancer in Africa. There is a direct connection between selenium levels in the soil of Senegal and the health of the people who live there. There are doctors and health care practitioners in Africa who are now using selenium supplementation along with other nutrients, to stop the progression of AIDS and to rebuild immune function. (AIDS is not present when the immune system is functioning normally.) According to the facts I have just presented about HIV/ AIDS, AIDS cannot develop when healthy selenium levels are maintained in someone who has the HIV virus.

Using ozone or hydrogen peroxide therapy and a nutritional approach to treat HIV/AIDS has been proven to be a safe, effective and inexpensive treatment for HIV/AIDS and many other diseases. It is my opinion that the current HIV/AIDS drug therapies do not compare, in any way, to the benefits of this natural approach. These natural non-drug therapies work quickly, effectively and safely! There are now a growing number of doctors around the world that say that HIV/AIDS can be cured through these methods.

In the past few years I have also seen news stories on the growing problem of antibiotic resistant bacterial infections and aggressive flesh eating bacterial infections. I believe the solution to these problems are ozone and hydrogen peroxide therapy. Ozone is more powerful than chlorine on bacteria cell walls and kills bacteria from 10 times to 3000 times faster than chlorine, depending on the concentration. I believe special nutritional supplementation should also be used. Not only are these therapies quickly effective in destroying hard to treat infections but they also increase oxygen levels in the body and boost natural immune function at the same time. What I would like to see is the media, medical and government officials begin to promote these therapies to deal with the many worldwide health problems that we are facing today.

CHAPTER 20

THE HEALTH CARE CRISIS

The health care crisis in our nation is being perpetuated by four basic things

1. The profit influence in our health care system

2. The FDA and government

3. The food industry

4. The ignorance of the people

In this discussion I recognize there are many people in the health care industry that are caring, genuine and experts in their field. This book is aimed at the people in the health care industry that know what they're doing is not the best care available but the most profitable. Health care professionals, such as doctors, should be true to the Hippocratic Oath, to their fellow man and to their creator.

Because of the greed and coercion in the pharmaceutical industry and other special interests in our health care system, that has gone on for so many years, our economy and the wealth of the American people is being hurled toward economic disaster. These industries have taken the wealth of the American people by fraud, bribery and coercion. The blood of the people is on their hands. How many people have died in this nation over the past 60+ years because of the failure of the FDA to serve the interests of the people rather than the interests of the pharmaceutical and health care industry? **It's time for things to change for the good of the people!**

We should look to other countries that have better health care systems that allow alternative therapies like ozone therapy. This is largely due to the fact that these governments don't cater to the special interests of the pharmaceutical and health care industries. Their health care systems are geared toward healing and actual cures!

After years of personal research on the subject of health care, it is my opinion that if our health care system were to focus on only the best and most effective therapies available, for the treatment of disease, it would become primarily a natural and holistic centered health care system. We would adopt dietary, nutritional and healthy lifestyle changes along with bio-oxidative therapies to be our primary medicines. If our health care system were to take this direction, the eventual outcome would mean saving hundreds of billions in health care costs in a relatively short period of time! **Cancer, heart disease, HIV/AIDS and many other diseases would be considered cured and conquered!**

There are many books and documentaries on the subject of the problems with our health care system. One of the best documentary's I've seen is called "Cancer-The Forbidden Cures." It details the many natural cures that have been used successfully over time to cure cancer, but one by one, they have been systematically rejected by our mainstream conventional health care system in favor of the expensive and harmful treatments that have been used for many years. You can buy the DVD on websites like Amazon or you can watch most of it on YouTube for free.

CHAPTER 21

CHILDHOOD HEALTH CARE

It seems in this modern age that we are living in we are seeing more childhood health problems than ever before. The health care industry is also growing along with these problems. As a person drives through major cities you can see huge new medical complexes being built including those designated just for children. According to the American Society of Clinical Oncology, cancer is the leading cause of childhood death in the U.S with 13,500 new diagnoses each year. Here are some of the other childhood diseases on the rise

ADHD

Allergy

Asthma

Asperger syndrome

Autism

Childhood obesity

Cystic fibrosis

Down syndrome

Diabetes

Muscular dystrophy

Muscular sclerosis

   Perhaps you've seen ads for children's charities or children's hospitals where children are given special attention and maybe even free medical care. You see the picture of the young child looking pale and with no hair because of the chemotherapy treatments they are receiving. I think any organization that reaches out to children is doing something great but the question is are they doing the right thing? In short, I believe chemotherapy is exactly the wrong thing to do to a child or any person if you want to see them get well.

   Our health care system has gotten way out of control. There is no universal standard or protocol in our health care system for determining the cause of a particular disease before a treatment is recommended or administered.

   Imagine a child is brought into a doctor's office for a checkup or for the doctor to look at a growth or bump. The doctor does an examination and then takes a biopsy. The lab results say its cancer. The child is put on chemotherapy for a period of time. After a number of months the doctor discovers the child's immune system has collapsed because of the chemotherapy. The cancer then begins to spread throughout the body. A few months later the child dies. The bill for these treatments could equal tens of thousands or even a hundred thousand dollars. If families really understood the odds of a child beating cancer through chemotherapy along with all of the long term side effects, I think most people would look for other options. I think the problem is a lot of people don't know there are other options and are not told about them.

Our health care system has taken, what I believe to be very simple issues, and made them incredibly complex and expensive, building a huge industry of all kinds of medical care that often only expands the problem rather than actually solving it.

Here is an example of one cause of disease. Most people would agree that with our modern farming techniques and all of the junk food that's out there today, that kids and even parents are not getting all of the necessary nutrients they need. As I mentioned earlier, there are places in the world where people don't get enough selenium because the soil is selenium deficient. (Selenium is a key necessary nutrient you cannot live without.) Then there are other places in the world where the soil is particularly rich in selenium and there is a direct connection to much lower rates of disease in these places. In the scenario I described above of the child being diagnosed with cancer and dying, imagine that this one particular child was not getting enough selenium in his diet which resulted in the growth forming on his body. The right solution to this particular child's health issue would be to determine the nutritional deficiency and correct it. To prescribe a proven selenium supplement along with healthy lifestyle and dietary changes. Through time the body would be able to shrink the tumor itself. Prescribing chemotherapy not only did not solve this child's problem but actually made it much worse in a short period of time, resulting in the child's death.

In the modern world that we live in there are lots of problems with people's diets, lifestyles and living and working environments. These are the first places we should be looking for the cause of disease. Nowadays we are surrounded by manmade synthetic materials, chemicals and volatile organic chemicals that the average person never thinks twice about. VOC'S can be coming out of many kinds of building materials including particle board underlayment. In can come from carpeting. It can come from cleaning chemicals and the residue left behind after cleaning. Books have been written on the health effects of synthetic materials and chemicals in different kinds of clothing. You can be exposed to harmful VOC'S at work every day depending upon what you do for a living. We can even be exposed to toxins coming from within our own bodies such as the mercury content in Amalgam dental fillings. Some people are more sensitive to these things and some people are not, but it's necessary to be aware of the pollutants you are being exposed to and consider the risk of becoming sick as a result of your exposure to these chemicals. In a home you can control many of these things by replacing synthetics with natural materials and cleaning with natural cleaners. It is my belief that many children are being adversely affected by these kinds of pollutants. One child may not have a problem while another may be particularly sensitive to certain pollutants and chemicals. In regard to the potential harm from amalgam fillings, it amazes me that they are still being used today when there is a better, safer alternative with composite fillings. Composite fillings are not only free of mercury but also affix better and look better.

When I was a Bible College student I had a class where the teacher was talking to us about the importance of coming together for church and sharing our prayer requests with one another. He related a story of a husband and wife at his church who requested prayer for their infant son who was very sick. Their child had a very serious case of diarrhea and it had gone on for so long their doctor expressed his concern it could stunt his growth. After they shared their request for prayer, a church member asked them a few questions and said he knew what the problem was. They were using tap water to mix their baby formula. The municipal water in that area was not good quality for drinking. They began mixing their formula with purified water and this serious and mysterious health problem was suddenly solved. It's interesting to note that their doctor did not have the solution. It is my whole hearted conviction that this sort of thing happens every day where there is a simple solution to people's health problems. Often times a person will seek medical help for a condition and our current health care system will look everywhere but the simplest and most likely place for the answer. The case about conventional cancer care is a perfect example.

Our health care system is also going in the wrong direction in regard to childhood vaccinations. I have read articles in recent years that stated that children now receive anywhere from 21 to more than 30 vaccinations in the first 16 months of life. In the last 40 years the number of childhood vaccinations has increased dramatically, and has doubled since 1991. This is particularly beneficial for the pharmaceutical companies that manufacture these vaccines, but the truth is we are toxifying and poisoning our children. This large number of vaccinations are actually creating a whole new set of problems in health care in regard to the long term effects they are having on children's health. As time passes there are an increasing number of doctors and researchers who are linking the mercury content, aluminum hydroxide and other ingredients in vaccines to a dramatic rise in neurological disorders in children, including autism, since 1991. There has been a rise in many other health problems as well.

I'm aware that the creation of certain vaccines, such as the polio vaccine, have been credited with virtually wiping out certain diseases from entire nations that once caused widespread and lifelong health problems. **However, there is such a thing as overkill.** That's what's happening today in America and other developed nations. There have been in depth, medically recognized studies done on this issue. There have also been a number of books written on this subject that clearly show the link between numerous infant immunizations and SIDS (Sudden Infant Death Syndrome.) Also a clear link has been established between numerous infant immunizations and many other health problems including the many neurological disorders we are seeing today. Here are two books on this subject by Dr. Viera Scheibner, "Vaccination: 100 Years of Orthodox Research Shows Vaccinations are a Medical Assault on the Immune System" and "Behavioral Problems in Childhood: The Link to Vaccination." Also there are a couple of websites, Mercola.com and GreenMedInfo that have many excellent in depth articles about the problems with past vaccines, current vaccines and potential vaccine use in coming years.

After reading some of these studies it's clear that the pharmaceutical companies who produce these vaccines, and the public health officials who make the policies for administering them, are completely aware of these serious medical issues. Yet it seems nothing changes in these public policies. Perhaps these people only view the children who die and who are crippled as just numbers or statistics. However, these children are not statistics to their parents and family. I think public policy would change if some of these people who are responsible for vaccination policy would, for a moment, put themselves in the shoes of the families who have been affected negatively by having their infant child die from SIDS or become crippled for life. Imagine the emotion and heart break of parents who have spent so much time and expense preparing for the arrival of their new child, only to be devastated by the loss of this child. Now they must prepare for their child's funeral. They invested so much time, emotion and expense, such as medical bills for the arrival of their new child. Now they must bear the emotional and financial cost of the funeral and burial of this same child. How would the people who administer these policies feel if this was their own child or grandchild? It would be a heart breaking and a completely avoidable tragedy.

One thing I think people need to realize about contagious diseases in developed nations like the U.S is that our health and health care standards have come a long way since the last great epidemic. In addition to this we also have much more knowledge about how to treat disease and build the immune system through natural means. Our health care system should focus more on building strong immune systems through natural, safer means the way the creator intended.

We should also be using ozone and hydrogen peroxide therapies as well.

Nutritional Therapy

Children born with Downs syndrome and other health issues should receive proven nutritional therapy from the time they are born, to make it possible for them to experience more normal development, since these conditions are often due to prenatal nutritional deficiency and the fact that infants and small children are still going through significant developmental change.

In the case of Downs Syndrome where there is an imbalance on the 21st chromosome, researchers have discovered that children with Downs Syndrome do not assimilate nutrients from their food like normal children. Because of their poor absorption of the nutrients in their food, Downs Syndrome children are actually suffering from a form of malnutrition. They require specialized nutrition. Dixie Lawrence, who appeared on ABC'S Nightline in December of 1996 shared her story of how she researched this subject for her adopted daughter Madison, who has Downs Syndrome. Through research, that eventually included blood tests to show actual nutrient levels in the blood, she formulated her own customized nutritional supplementation. Shortly after starting Madison on her new nutritional regimen she observed that it brought about dramatic improvements in Madison's behavioral development. Dixie went on to work with a company to produce a nutritional product, based on her original formula, for Downs Syndrome children. This product which is now available is called Nutrivene-D which, according to one article I read, is now being used by more than 15,000 children.

CHAPTER 22

OTHER DISEASES

As I mentioned in the beginning of my book, this edition is not intended to be an exhaustive resource on every disease or health issue but to give you some important basic insights. There are a lot of diseases I haven't covered such as diabetes, Parkinson's disease, multiple sclerosis, muscular dystrophy and so on. However, the main thing that I believe all of these diseases have in common is that we see them happening in our modern society with all of our modern processed foods, food additives and chemicals and pollution in our air and water. Conversely we see that indigenous people groups in other parts of the world, that are still eating their natural native diets, do not have these diseases. They remain physically active in the fresh air and sunshine and are eating whole natural unprocessed foods. When we bring the body into nutritional and chemical balance and free it from harmful chemicals and pollution, it is then that the body can begin to reverse disease and return to its natural state of health. There are many excellent holistic doctors and nutritionists out there with a wealth of knowledge and experience who cover these other diseases in greater detail than I do in this book. Once again I would like to encourage you to take the time do your own research and read after the doctors and experts I have mentioned in this book. Here are some other resources: The Weston Price Foundation, Georgia Janisch R.D and Mercola.com. Mercola.com by Dr. Joseph Mercola has the largest volume of alternative medicine articles that I have seen so far. There are many other well-known health experts and holistic doctors out there, too many for me to list. Not all of these health experts necessarily agree with one another on every issue, for example some are 100% against soy while others say some soy products have value or some soy products are safe and some are not. You have to take some time to read up on these issues and specific products and come to your own conclusions. Take time to seek out the wisdom of God on these issues and for your life.

CHAPTER 23

THE GREAT AMERICAN HEALTH CARE COVER UP

As I have presented in this book, there are certain entities within our health care establishment, that have purposely and systematically worked, through lobbying, coercion, and fraud to keep certain alternative treatments out of main stream medicine for many years, for the sake of market control and profits.

These entities, such as the pharmaceutical industry, the American Medical Association and the FDA, through their efforts have purposely resisted natural non-patentable cures and in place have given us many therapies and procedures that are inferior and even harmful and hopeless.

A number of years ago I had a dream. In this dream I was in a hallway looking at an indoor pool and a vestibule that led to the pool, with glass walls and glass doors. The lighting was dim. People who were ill were in the vestibule, waiting for their opportunity to get to the waters of the pool. The pool was covered with a sheet of clear plastic and holding the plastic in place were giant flies. The people in the vestibule area were very sick. Some were dying and some were already dead. They could not get to the pool.

Like in the Biblical account of the pool of Bethesda, the waters in the pool represented healing. The healing was there but was being obstructed and withheld from the people. The giant flies represent spiritual influences preventing the people from being healed. The main spiritual influences represented by the flies are greed, selfishness and the love of money. These things were the spiritual down fall of the rich man, in the Biblical account of the rich man and the beggar Lazarus, in Luke 16:19-31. The rich man ended up going to hell because he had no compassion for the suffering beggar, who was laid at the rich man's gate, who was covered with sores and eventually died. The rich man could have easily helped the beggar but counted the beggar an unimportant person, not realizing he was forsaking his own mercy as well!

This dream represents much of what is happening in our health care system today. Every year more than one million Americans die from cancer and heart disease alone! This does not include all of the people currently suffering from cancer and heart disease. This does not include all of the other diseases that Americans suffer from and die from annually.

Here is another dream I had about health care roughly 20 years ago. After 20 years I still remember this dream clearly because it was a spiritual dream, an inspired dream from God. In the dream I was on a beach in Upper Michigan. It was just south of where the Cedar River flows out to Green Bay. In the dream I looked out at the beautiful golden beach in amazement. Then I looked down at the sand and saw what looked like a small stream flowing beneath my feet under the sand. Somehow I was able to see through the sand. I noticed what looked like a white cell flowing in the stream that was about the size of a small apricot. I reached down to touch it and when I did it turned a dark blue. When I withdrew my finger it changed back to white. With a gentle touch the cell went through a dramatic change and then turned back again to its original state. Then I saw a man on the beach with a rototiller turning and churning up everything I had just seen. This man was a medical doctor.

Here is the meaning of the dream. The beach represents the human body. God created it perfect and beautiful. The stream under the beach represents the blood stream and the white cell was a cell in the blood stream. My touch and the changing color of the cell revealed how the body is designed to respond to a soft touch of intervention. Through right dietary and lifestyle changes the body responds with health and correct function. The rototiller that the doctor was using to mix everything up, represents what medical science often does when it uses drugs and surgery to try to correct problems with the body. Instead of bringing the body back into biochemical and nutritional balance they often create greater chemical confusion in the body without offering a real cure.

Once again this dream represents much of what is going on in our health care system today, in regard to the treatment of chronic disease, where there is a lot of things being done for profit sake while true cures are being systematically avoided or withheld. If it could be proven that such coercion and conspiracy have occurred in the FDA and our medical establishment over the last 60 to 70 years and that true cures have been withheld from the people, then certain entities within our health care system and the pharmaceutical industry could be found guilty of such crimes. As a result, they could be made to pay restitution that could equal billions of dollars in health care damages. Ozone therapy and other natural therapies being taken away from the American people in the early years of the FDA are examples in this case.

Here is another example of what I'm talking about. How many times do we see ads asking for support for cancer research, breast cancer research, childhood cancer research, muscular dystrophy and many other diseases? We see these ads often and all over the place. **Here is what most people don't realize; the people who are doing the research are not looking for a cure, they are looking for a pharmaceutical cure if they are really looking for a cure at all.** The real cures for these diseases are already here! The cures are found in nature and in the human body. The problem with this is that natural cures are generally not patentable treatments and therefore are not profitable, or not as profitable, as patented drug therapies like statin or chemotherapy drugs for example.

Modern Medicine, Let The Buyer Beware

After everything that I have said about our health care system that is negative, I do believe that there are valuable things being done also, however it is ultimately up to the patient, the consumer, to do their own research before electing to receive a specific treatment or surgery. If every patient or patients' family would take the time to do their own research of the different options available, in main stream medicine and alternative medicine, our health care system would have been forced to change long ago for the better.

CHAPTER 24

THE AFFORDABLE CARE ACT

I began writing this book back in 2011 before a lot of issues came to light about the so called Affordable Care Act. From the onset there have been many people who have been either adamantly for or against it. People who are for it believe in it because it's supposed make health care available to every citizen regardless of income or current health. People who are against it believe it is increasing the federal governments powers over our individual rights and civil liberties and even forcing citizens to support things that go against their moral and spiritual beliefs. In addition, to their dismay, people have also discovered that many of the promises made about the ACA, also known as Obama Care, did not materialize. For those in the middle class, many have found it significantly more expensive than their previous insurance. I personally know of one middle class family of four that is looking at a premium increase of almost three times what they previously had been paying. Many people also discovered they were not able to keep the same insurance or the same doctor as was promised.

One of the biggest problems of this new law is the enormity of it. The PPACA, HCERA and the final regulations are more than 10,500 pages long. Some have estimated that the regulations alone consist of more than 11 million words. I believe that 99.99 percent of Americans do not understand the majority of what is contained in this law and the additional powers granted to the federal government through it. In other words, people are losing certain freedoms that they do not even know about.

Now there are some experts who are saying that they believe the ACA was never created to succeed. That the Obama administrations goal is to use the ACA as a stepping stone to bring in a single payer nationalized health care system. Such a system would dramatically increase the power of the federal government and take away more of our freedoms. In other words, everyone who is above the poverty line would have to pay into this system through increases in taxes but what individual citizens get in return, in terms of health care, is in the hands of a bureaucratic system.

Those who oppose nationalized health care argue that it grants the central government the ultimate control over the population. That if leaders wanted to engage in population control this would be the vehicle by which to do it. Vladimir Lenin, the first premier of the Soviet Union, has been quoted as saying "Socialized medicine is the keystone to the arch of the socialist state." Today's reality is that population growth in the world is becoming an ever increasing concern to world leaders including those who do not believe in Gods purpose for the earth. In fact, this is probably the number one concern among secular humanists apart from climate change. Secular humanists, rather than viewing people as Gods children, view the masses as little more than cattle, including non-producing eaters that just use up space and resources. They believe the best way to solve the world's problems is to reduce the world population to a manageable number. Such a plan, in their view, would solve the problem of pollution, global warming and save the earth from the destruction being caused by man. However, God has a better plan and purpose and that is to save man, but it is up to us to believe in Gods plans and purposes and to look to him. Gods view is that every person matters, every individual is important and was created for a purpose.

In the times we are living in people often talk about issues relating to end time prophecy, the book of Revelation and the appearance of the antichrist. Throughout history there have been many antichrist types. We see in the scriptures that among the main goals of the antichrist is to create a one world government and to control the masses. Why does God permit this to occur? Because of an unbelieving world. Because of the unbelief of man and the selfishness of man. If the world turned to God, believed in his word and looked for the return of Christ, no antichrist would ever come into power. Gods perfect will would be permitted to go forward in the earth. What is Gods perfect will? To believe in him and to love one another even as he has loved us. To do unto others as you would have done unto you. To fulfill the law of Christ.

From the standpoint of someone who does not agree with the ACA, the issue of making health care available and affordable to everyone is a very real issue but it has also been a great political selling point for the politicians who support the ACA and want to garner votes from it. (At least up until recently.) However, what they didn't tell you is the hidden agendas that are behind it.

The number one problem I see with socialized health care from the standpoint of human compassion and making health care available to all citizens, is the double standards and conflicts of interests at the highest levels of government. **If government leaders cared as much for its citizens as they say they do, wouldn't they first seek to remove the treatments and therapies that are not working and legalize and support those that do?** After all, what good is free or low cost health care if it harms you or ends up killing you? I believe focusing on the best treatments and therapies would be the best way to begin health care reform along with the creation of legislation that would help to set price limits. Prices that are in line with the current cost of living as we see done in other countries where health care is far more affordable. Perhaps prices based on actual profit margin percentages or lower prices through better competition in the market place. Part of this would have to involve tort reform. If our federal government supported the best health care options that currently exist, with creating some type of price controls, health care and health care insurance would be affordable to the average citizen without the ACA. In addition, the government would be able to afford to cover those who cannot afford health care through Medicaid and other programs. Everyone would be insurable because everyone would be curable!

Some would argue that there are other nations like the U.K and Canada that have had successful nationalized health care for years. There are people in these countries who have had positive experiences getting the health care they needed. However, there are others who haven't. Sometimes people are put on long waiting lists for procedures they can't afford to wait for or their age puts them into a bracket where it's no longer considered cost effective to provide certain procedures or therapies. Those people, if they have the money, will end up going elsewhere to get the health care they need and pay for it themselves. If they can't afford to go elsewhere, they may suffer or die while waiting for their appointment or because they no longer qualify because of age. Those people who go elsewhere are not only paying for their health care through taxes but they end up paying privately out of pocket as well.

As we have seen with the mountain of regulations in the ACA and the projected cost of implementing it is that running health care through a bureaucratic system is expensive and inefficient. The one thing that nationalized health care does well is it puts the entire health care system in the control of the central government. Doing this is taking a step toward a socialistic or even communistic state. It does not represent the independent or free market system of America. It promotes dependence rather than independence. The great thing about promoting independence in a nation is that people are required to think and work for what they have. They learn how to take responsibility for things. When a country promotes an attitude of dependence in any area, people begin to forget how to do things. Then when there is a collapse in a major state run system that everyone has become dependent on, you end up with a major catastrophe where people feel helpless and are in peril. Consider the results of a failure in a major electric grid or water system. Everything in that area becomes paralyzed except for those who have backup systems in place. Consider the failure of an entire economic system such as the

Soviet Union, where every citizen was dependent on the central government for virtually everything! The history of the Soviet Union is a proven model of what ultimately occurs in a totally dependent society. We also see the same example being played out in North Korea.

What we need is honesty and transparency in our government and an end to the secret deals made behind closed doors between politicians and big business. What our nation needs is to return to faith in God and in his word. Personally I'd rather live in a cabin in the back woods and live off the land rather than be a partaker of a corrupt system that takes advantage of other people. In other words, a person who is benefiting from secret deals in government. At least in the back woods I'd have a clear conscience that I haven't done anyone wrong. You can't put a price on the value of knowing you did what was right. However, realistically we all need to be involved in our government for the purpose of positive change and accountability.

CHAPTER 25

A WORD FOR THE RICH

The Bible has a lot to say about the rich that is not positive because the rich have a tendency to focus on self-sufficiency, power and materialism rather than God. In America we see this truth played out to an extreme level in corporate America and in the pharmaceutical and health care industries. There is such enormous wealth out there in these areas that these industries have had the power to shape large segments of our entire health care system for the purpose of profit making. As we look into the scriptures we see that money and power are not the most important things but the state of the human heart and soul is the most important. Why is this? Because as we see in the scriptures we are only here for a little while and then we die. We pass from this life to the next and what do we get to take with us? We take with us the deeds we have done in this life, how we have treated our brothers and sisters, our fellow man. We must leave all worldly wealth and possessions behind. The only wealth we can take with us is the wealth we invest in the kingdom of God. The wealth we invest in Gods plans and purposes in the earth.

No man can serve two masters, for either he will hate the one and love the other, or he will be devoted to the one and despise the other. You cannot serve God and money. Matthew 6:24 (NIV)

This passage is saying we must choose which one has the highest priority in our life. Either we will serve God or we will serve money!

CHAPTER 26

THE GREAT PHYSICAN

The good news is that God can heal and restore the things that man cannot. Medically documented miracles happen every day! Even the spontaneous regeneration of organs and body parts have been medically documented! Christ is still The Great Physician! Here are some passages of scripture that have to do with divine healing.

He sent his word, and healed them... Psalm 107:20

The Spirit of the Lord is upon me, because he hath anointed me to preach the gospel to the poor; he hath sent me to heal the broken hearted, to preach deliverance to the captives, and recovering of sight to the blind, to set at liberty them that are bruised, To preach the acceptable year of the Lord. Luke 4:18-19

And great multitudes came unto him, having with them those that were lame, blind, dumb, maimed, and many others, and cast them down at Jesus' feet; and he healed them: Insomuch that the multitude wondered, when they saw the dumb to speak, the maimed to be whole, the lame to walk, and the blind to see: And they glorified the God of Israel. Matthew 15:30-31

And they came to Jericho: and as he went out of Jericho with his disciples and a great number of people, blind Bartimaeus, the son of Timaeus, sat by the highway side begging. And when he heard that it was Jesus of Nazareth, he began to cry out, and say, Jesus, thou son of David, have mercy on me. And many charged him that he should hold his peace: But he cried the more a great deal, thou son of David, have mercy on me. And Jesus stood still and commanded him to be called. And they call the blind man, saying unto him, Be of good comfort, rise; he calleth thee. And he, casting away his garment, rose, and came to Jesus. And Jesus answered and said unto him, What will thou that I should do unto thee? The blind man said unto him, Lord, that I might receive my sight. And Jesus said unto him, Go thy way; thy faith hath made thee whole. And immediately he received his sight, and followed Jesus in the way. Mark 10:46-52

. . . and healed all that were sick: That it might be fulfilled which was spoken by Isaiah the prophet, saying, Himself took our infirmities, and bare our sicknesses. Matthew 8:16-17

Is any sick among you? Let him call for the elders of the church; and let them pray over him, anointing him with oil in the name of the Lord: And the prayer of faith shall save the sick, and the Lord shall raise him up; and if he have committed sins, they shall be forgiven him. James 5:14-15

For verily I say unto you, That whosoever shall say unto this mountain, Be thou removed, and be thou cast into the sea;

and shall not doubt in his heart, but shall believe that those things which he saith shall come to pass; he shall have whatsoever he saith. Therefore I say unto you, What things soever ye desire, when ye pray, believe that ye receive them, and ye shall have them. Mark 11:23-24

CHAPTER 27

THE SIMPLICITY OF HEALTH CARE AND THE MYSTERY OF HEALTH AND HEALING

I believe the subject of effective health care is like a puzzle. Not a difficult puzzle but a simple one. We all learn about health issues over time. If a person is observant, through the course of time, you learn what foods seem to give the best health effect and what foods do not. We learn what kind of activities and exercise seem to give the best health results and which things don't. For example, when I'm doing physical work outside in the fresh air and sunshine, I feel and look much healthier than when I'm sitting in a chair doing office work all day. I feel much better and much healthier when I eat healthy whole foods, like an apple or whole grain bread, rather than a high sugar soft drink or dessert. Over time a person should gather knowledge from various sources so you can create a mental library of proven health care knowledge, of things that work and things that do not work. Things you should be doing and things you should avoid.

I guess it's true that there are people who can eat unhealthy food their whole life and think they are just fine, until they have a health crisis. I find this hard to relate to. Maybe I'm more observant than the average person. I found as a young person that when I ate junk food it ultimately made me feel like junk. I felt unsatisfied and unfulfilled as opposed to how you feel when you have a healthy, well rounded meal. I began to observe that I got the best health effect from eating healthy foods consistently throughout the day. In other words, don't skip meals and eat when you're hungry. There are a lot people who live their lives just scrapping by, health wise, who never really think about how their body works and what it's actually doing from day to day. They get up in the morning, look in the mirror, they see the same basic thing they saw yesterday. They eat the same stuff, do the same things, not realizing that their body is constantly producing new cells and new tissue. Your body is a tissue plant or factory. Your body is like a building made up of many different materials that require regular maintenance. If you use poor quality materials you're going to have a poor quality building. Your body is like a work horse built for all kinds of work. You harness its power by giving it the right nutrition and care.

In regard to the subject of disease, I believe the cures for most diseases are much simpler than people realize. As simple as making some simple lifestyle changes. As simple as making some dietary changes or even adding a single nutrient that you are deficient in. It's as simple as the quality of the water you drink and the air you breathe. Are you living and working in a healthy environment or one that's going to make you ill?

Also there is a spiritual aspect of life, which is really the most important because we see in the scriptures that the physical world came out of the spiritual world. God spoke and it was. When we take time to pray, read and meditate on the scriptures, when we learn to love and forgive, all of these are foundational issues that we must deal with to experience health and wellbeing from the inside out. Through the scriptures and from the Spirit of God we gain wisdom and understanding and most important of all we gain eternal life through faith in him and in his son.

When you put all of these pieces of the puzzle together in your own life, then you have succeeded in creating the whole picture of everything you must do to experience optimum health in your lifetime and in the lives of others that you share your knowledge with!

CHAPTER 28

The following is a letter I wrote in October of 2014 addressing the Ebola crisis in Africa. I sent the letter out to Christian pastors by email on October 24th 2014.

Ebola and "A Hypocritical Oath"

Several years ago I wrote a letter called "A Hypocritical Oath" which was about the problems with our health care and medical establishment here in America. In it I discussed how there are better treatments for certain diseases that are not being used in mainstream medicine, and that the best and most effective treatments are often passed over for ones that are more profitable but not as good.

Recently the outbreak of Ebola in West Africa has been in the news frequently. There has been a lot of talk about an experimental vaccine that has not yet been approved by the FDA. The thing that bothers me and many others, about the handling of this issue by our government and medical authorities, is it seems they offer no clear solutions or preventive actions that can be taken to help people avoid becoming sick, except for not coming in contact with infected individuals. I have noticed that advice about what people can do for themselves is coming from sources other than the government and medical authorities because our so called authorities are not putting forth such information.

Another thing that has bothered me about the Ebola outbreak is how little has been said about how Ebola patients are being treated. It seems only recently that some of this information has come out. I have read about how both Canada and China are planning to make new Ebola vaccines available soon. Recently I read an article from Rasta Livewire on how some Nigerian Doctors defeated Ebola with water! In other words, making sure patients stayed properly hydrated so their immune systems could fight the disease.

As I had written in my letter "A Hypocritical Oath," which I'm going to be publishing in book form, there is an area of medicine that our health care system in America has failed to use, while numerous other countries have. The area is that of bio-oxidative therapy or specifically, ozone and hydrogen peroxide therapy. Ozone and hydrogen peroxide have already been approved for sterilization and water purification. Ozone or O3, is being used widely, to safely and cheaply kill all pathogens in many commercial and municipal water treatment systems here in the U.S. Unlike the United States, there is a list of numerous other countries that have approved its use for medical purposes, including the purification of blood. It has been proven to be safe and effective and for good reason. The human immune system itself produces oxidative molecules such as hydrogen peroxide and ozone. Most people are aware of the disinfectant use of 3% hydrogen peroxide that is available at local drug stores, but very few people know that their immune system produces it for the same purpose, to kill infection. In other words, hydrogen peroxide is Gods cleanser and medicine of the body.

What sets ozone and hydrogen peroxide apart from other chemical agents is the way they work. The free radical oxygen atoms that are released from ozone and hydrogen peroxide tear through the thin cell walls of viral and bacterial infections. Human cell walls are thicker and more resistant. Ozone and hydrogen peroxide are also set apart because they are safe, inexpensive and have the ability to kill every pathogen known. Another very important benefit of using these therapies is that they improve circulation and oxygen levels in the blood and body tissues. It's a benefit that does not occur with heavy doses of antibiotic or antiviral drugs. Sometimes heavy doses of these drugs can dramatically reduce circulation of oxygenated blood and have severe health consequences. There can also be severe health consequences from vaccines as well, depending on what is in them and how an individual reacts to them.

I think that the medical community is doing a great disservice to mankind by not making greater use of this bio-oxidative area of medicine. Simple and inexpensive ozone generators could be used in third world nations simply by connecting them to small, inexpensive solar panel generators. Using hydrogen peroxide orally or intravenous drips would also be a simple and inexpensive way to treat individuals that have contracted Ebola and other diseases. Also, as I mentioned in the article from Nigeria, Professor Akin Osibogun stated that it is of key importance to keep the patient's hydration and electrolyte levels up since the disease causes severe dehydration. Keeping up proper hydration and electrolytes gives the patients own immune system the opportunity to fight the disease and overcome it.

If I was a health worker or doctor working with an at risk population, I would encourage people to take certain steps to boost their immune systems and boost their hydrogen peroxide levels. I would advise people to take the steps listed below.

*Take care of your health

*Get sufficient sleep

*Eat a healthy diet

*Take some quality nutritional supplements that include vitamin C with citrus bioflavonoids, selenium, Zinc, and vitamin D
(Higher doses of vitamin C will create higher levels of hydrogen peroxide in the blood.)

*Exercise

*Get fresh air and sunshine

*Drink plenty of purified water

*Maintain healthy electrolyte levels

*Maintain personal hygiene, like hand washing. (Something the Nigerian government has stressed since the outbreak.)

If a person is feeling ill, I would have them begin some type of ozone or hydrogen peroxide therapy.

I have found countless articles and studies on the subject of ozone and hydrogen peroxide therapy including simple protocols and dosages. I have even read a number of articles about how hydrogen peroxide was successfully used by British medical practitioners to save people's lives during the influenza outbreak of 1918-1920 in India. Incidentally the symptoms of influenza were very similar to those of Ebola.

I would also encourage prayer for those who are sick since the scriptures tell us the Lord is our healer. The scriptures also tell us God can give us wisdom on what we should be doing.

Here are some names of individuals who have done successful research with hydrogen peroxide therapy:

Father Richard R. Wilhelm (also known as Father hydrogen peroxide)

Dr. Maynard Murray

Dr. Martin Fischer

Dr. Reginold Holeman

Dr. Edward Carl Rosenow, who worked at the Mayo Clinic for 62 years.

Dr. Charles Farr

Dr. David G. Williams, who wrote an in-depth article entitled "The Many Benefits of Hydrogen Peroxide."

Unfortunately, there are some hurdles that have to be overcome to using ozone and hydrogen peroxide more widely for medical purposes. The main hurdle is convincing doctors and governments that this is a worthwhile area to pursue amid resistance from the pharmaceutical industry. Even if these bio-oxidative therapies were used widely, I don't believe it would do away with the vaccine or antibiotic industries. It would just add another avenue of treatment to help people who may not have any other options. As I mentioned in my letter "A Hypocritical Oath" it is the duty of every doctor who has taken the Hippocratic Oath to make the patients welfare their first priority and use every avenue available to heal the patient. There is no amount of monetary gain that has greater value than having a clear conscience that an individual has done all that they can do to help save the life of another person.

Here is my opinion. If our health care authorities were really doing their best to serve the good of the people, this kind of information would and should become common knowledge to the general public.

Sincerely,
Rev. James Hogan

Update on Ebola Treatment

Recently, this year, 2015, I did an internet search on the subject of Ebola and ozone therapy. I came across several articles written by Dr. Mercola. One article was from October 26th 2014 titled Ozone Therapy: A possible Answer to Ebola? Another one was from January 4th 2015 entitled Updates on Ebola and ozone therapy. In the second article Dr. Mercola discusses an interview he had with Dr. Robert Rowen on the topic of ozone therapy for Ebola patients in Africa. Dr. Robert Rowen is a recognized leading expert in the U.S on bio-oxidative therapies. In October of 2014 the President of Sierra Leone invited Dr. Rowen to bring his team there to teach Sierra Leone doctors and health care workers how to administer ozone therapy on Ebola patients. Dr. Howard Robins who created the Robins method and protocols using Direct Intravenous Ozone Gas Administration (DIV) was also present. (The gas used is 99% oxygen and 1% ozone.) Dr. Rowen agreed and traveled with his team to Sierra Leone along with all kinds of medical equipment that was donated for the trip. After they had taken all of the time and trouble to train the doctors and health care workers, a call came from the assistant minister of health and then the minister of health himself, that there would be no ozone treatments administered to individuals with Ebola. You can read the entire article on Mercola.com and you can also watch the interview on You Tube.

Why were experimental drugs allowed to be used in Sierra Leone during the Ebola crisis but something like ozone, which has long been proven safe and effective, strictly denied? It's not difficult to figure out. We must assume the influence of money was the reason, either from the pharmaceutical industry and or from those who had paid positions to oversee the Ebola crisis in Sierra Leone. If there was influence from the pharmaceutical industry I think people must conclude that this kind of influence and persuasion is no different than that of an illegal drug cartel and also is in violation of antitrust laws. It should be considered a crime against mankind. At the very least bio-oxidative therapies should be allowed to compete on an equal footing with other therapies.

In a more recent article Dr. Rowen explained they did have the opportunity to treat five individuals that had become symptomatic. All five had their disease reversed within hours. He said this event was never acknowledged by the media in Sierra Leone. Dr. Rowen also stated that all of the medical equipment they brought there for treating Ebola was left there for the doctors and health workers to use. Dr. Mercola stated that in December of 2014 the New England Journal of Medicine reported a steady decrease in mortality rates of Ebola patients in the Hastings area of Sierra Leone from late September up to December 7th where they had decreased from 47.7% to 23.4%. Dr. Rowen commented that ozone may have continued to be used there after his departure.

A Prayer for Salvation

Do you know where you will go when you die? Would you like to find peace with God in your life? This is the reason why Jesus came to earth. He came tell us about Gods love and eternal kingdom. He came to a fallen world with the gospel message; the message of good news that we can be reconciled to God through him. Jesus came to be the mediator between a holy God and a fallen and sinful world. He came to bring us new life and he came to heal us also. Jesus came to invite us to be members of the family of God. We receive these things by faith because they are spiritual and they are spiritually discerned. We simply say "Lord, I believe and I receive."

Romans 10:9-13

If you confess with your mouth the Lord Jesus and believe in your heart that God has raised Him from the dead, you will be saved. For with the heart one believes unto righteousness, and with the mouth confession is made unto salvation. For the Scripture says, "Whoever believes on Him will not be put to shame." For there is no distinction between Jew and Greek, for the same Lord over all is rich to all who call upon Him. For "whoever calls on the name of the LORD shall be saved."

You can pray a simple pray like this:

Dear Heavenly Father, I come to you in the name of your son Jesus. I believe Jesus died for my sins and rose again from the dead, that I may be saved. Forgive me of my sins. I invite you into my heart. Thank you Heavenly Father for giving me new life through Jesus and for inviting me to spend eternity in Heaven with you forever. Amen.

I would like to encourage you to take time to know God through his word, the Bible, and through prayer daily. I would also like to encourage you to find a church, a place of Christian fellowship, where you can grow in your faith and be part of a body of believers who can encourage you and support you in your daily faith walk. In addition, I've always believed that the local church is the best place to network with other people to help us in all areas of life.

Bibliography

New King James Version. Thomas Nelson and Sons, New York, New York, 1982. (NKJV)

New International Version of the Holy Bible. Zondervan Bible. Publishers, Grand Rapids, 1978. (NIV)

www.ingramcontent.com/pod-product-compliance
Lightning Source LLC
Chambersburg PA
CBHW070250190526
45169CB00001B/358